painful yarns*

metaphors &
stories to help
understand
the biology of
pain.

by

g. lorimer moseley

*yarn:\'yärn\, *noun,* a tale, especially a
story of adventure or incredible
happenings <He told a ripping good yarn>

To buy this book, go to any good bookshop. It would be cheaper to go to:

www.lulu.com

www.physiouk.co.uk

This edition of painful yarns is published in 2007 by Dancing Giraffe Press.

A CiP catalogue record for this title is available from the National Library of Australia:

Moseley, G. Lorimer (Graham Lorimer) 1970-
    Painful yarns. Metaphors & stories to help understand the biology of pain.

    Bibliography.
    Includes index.
    ISBN 9780980358803 (pbk.)

    1. pain – fiction. 2. Pain – Physiological aspects – fiction. 3. Rehabilitation – Fiction. I. Title.
    A823.4

This book uses Century Gothic 8 pt font, *Bell MT italic 12 pt font*, & Eurostile 11 pt font. Printed & bound in Spain by Lulu.com.

Front cover: A French bakery. Photograph by Stephen A. Edwards, New York, NY, USA.

Back cover: Pleasure or pain? Photograph by Kaboobi3, Oxford, UK.

This book should be cited as: Moseley, GL (2007) Painful yarns. Metaphors & stories to help understand the biology of pain. Dancing Giraffe Press. Canberra, Australia: 113 pages.

~ dancing giraffe press ~

Contents

List of figures

introduction

I decided to write this book after a great deal of lobbying from two groups of people. The first group was patients with whom I shared these stories as I tried to explain to them what we now know about the biology of pain. I love stories as a way to back up biology. I am convinced that if people in pain can understand their pain in terms of its underlying biology, it helps them cope with it and ultimately overcome it. I rely on *Explain Pain*[Ref List No. 1] to present the biology, and I use stories like the ones in this book to 'cement' it. So this book is for people in pain.

The second group who lobbied for this book was clinicians with whom I shared some of these stories at conferences, at seminars and at courses. I would always get asked 'Have you written those stories down?' Well, now I have. I have read versions of some of these stories being recounted as part of pain management program manuals. I am cool with that, but I didn't feel right about the way the stories had become that little bit grander than they already were – I think one had me flying a helicopter while half conscious (I didn't rush to correct it mind you – I felt a bit like Skippy the Bush Kangaroo). So, this book is for clinicians.

I have three hopes for this book. First, I hope you find the stories as interesting and as fun as I do. Second, I hope the stories help you understand the biology of pain. Third, I hope that TMBA, Mick, JK, Frank, Heidi, Smurph, Davo, Hannu, Dimos & Tan know I really appreciate your comments and suggestions on earlier versions of painful yarns.

Lorimer, Oxford, 2007.

4

nigel's superskoda 110

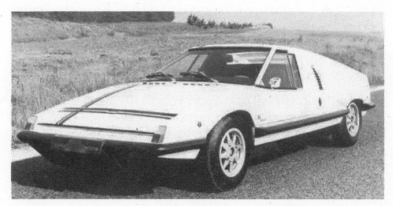

Or: Pain is a critical protective
device. Ignore it at your own peril.

When I first left school, I got what remains the coolest job I have ever had. It was so cool, I can't even write here where I worked, nor what exactly I did. Now *that* is cool. I *can* say, however, that Nigel Mawson worked there too.

5

Nigel was the nicest of about 15 middle aged investigative coppers[1]. They were hard men. Nigel was a hard man too, there is no doubt about that, but he was a South Australian and sounded a bit like David Hookes. David Hookes was a cricketer[2] who once told me I had a good straight drive but I needn't try and hit the cover off the ball. That David Hookes said I had a good straight drive was enough for me, as a 14 year old, to like him. That Nigel Mawson sounded like him was enough for me, as a 19 year old, to like *him*.

The other thing that was peculiar and, to me, a bit endearing, was that he had an unusual habit of referring to everyone by their full name. I was always Lorimer Moseley. Never Lorimer. Never Moseley. Always Lorimer Moseley. He also did this in the third person - "I will be taking Lorimer Moseley out with me today – there is something Lorimer Moseley ought to see". I have always been drawn to people who adhere to a silly little habit like that, even when to do so is considered by everyone else to be undoubtedly odd. So, unlike the rest of the grim-faced, overweight, estranged-from-their-family, married-to-their-job, chain smoking, heavy drinking blokes, Nigel didn't scare me. That is why one day I asked him for a lift home from work.

Nigel drove a 1971 Skoda SuperSport 110. Nigel didn't care for it, particularly. In fact, he made it clear that he refused to know anything at all about cars, simply because his brother had always been obsessed by them. Nigel said that as teenagers, his brother was as obsessed with cars as Nigel was with girls. He said:

> *Nigel Mawson: "My brother would want to get busy with his girl in the back of his car so he could check out how his CAR performed! He used to sit outside the loo while I was in there reading MAD magazines. I'd shove loo paper in ears to avoid hearing him carry on about*

---

1 Coppers: Police officers.
2 Cricket: Cricket is a sport played throughout the British Commonwealth.

needing to bore out[3] *my Datsun 180B, and that my mates were all uncool because none of them had extractors."*

Nigel's brother had the last laugh however, by leaving Nigel the Skoda in his will.

The Skoda SuperSport 110 was a magnificently ridiculous car. The doors didn't shut properly. The ignition only started if the right hand indicator was on. It leaked in the rain and sounded like a kettle the very second it hit 51 mph. The most striking thing however, was not about the car. No, the most striking thing was this; before starting the car, Nigel would turn on the radio, detune it so there was nothing but static, and then turn it up to maximum volume. Only then would he start the car up.

There was no point attempting conversation once the radio was on. One day, I asked him before we got in:

LM: "Nigel Mawson, why do you have the radio up so loud and why don't you ever tune it? Why don't you listen to <u>something</u> *instead of that terrible static?"*

NM: "It's not that loud Lorimer Moseley."

LM: "Oh but it is Nigel Mawson, it is."

NM: "I suppose I did think the horn was busted the other day because I couldn't hear it over the radio. I have the radio on to get rid of a strange knocking noise this car has. I hate knocking noises."

---

3 To bore out: To 'bore out' means to make the engine's cylinders a bit wider so as to turn a 2000 cc engine into a 2200 cc engine. Extractors do something to make the exhaust come out of the engine more efficiently – they 'extract' the air. Somehow. The side effect is that they make the car sound a bit chunkier. My mate Stevie put extractors on his VW beetle because he reckoned it made it sound like an RX-7. I reckon it sounded like a food processor.

LM (bemused and only vaguely interested look on face): "Right"

NM: "Yeah, about a month after I got the little shitbox, a year or so ago I guess, I noticed a little tapping noise, somewhere at the front there (Nigel waved a disinterested hand toward the front of the car). *It went away when I turned on the radio, so I didn't think more about it. The radio has somethin' wrong with it so that every time I get in here I have to turn it up again. Then the radio went completely jiggered and had basically no volume - I could hear the tapping noise something fierce in the gaps between sentences or songs. So I shifted the tuning a bit and that seemed to do the trick."*

LM: "So what was- what is, the noise?"

NM: "Fucked if I know. Fucked if I care."

LM: "You are a very interesting man Nigel Mawson"

NM: "And you are a prying little prick Lorimer Moseley"

I learnt fairly early on to not take such insults as if they are meant to mean what they say. With Nigel, and most of the people with whom I worked, such insults were rather complimentary. Nigel was right about the noise – as soon as he started the engine up, I couldn't hear a thing. Although I could feel it. I could feel the whole car thumping from side to side. The Skoda *felt* like it would break apart any minute. I must have looked a little surprised because Nigel shouted over the radio fuzz:

NM: "She's a bit rough. Sit on your coat, stick your feet on that wine cask and wedge your arm in under that bar – that way you'll hardly notice it."

8

So, I sat on my coat, put my feet on the wine cask and wedged my arm in under the bar. It all but concealed the violence of the bump and now it just felt like we were on a flat bottom raft in choppy seas. Nigel was certainly satisfied and we drove toward my house in silence. Except the radio.

My house was at the bottom of a dead-end street, the entrance to which had a little kerb. Typical middle class suburbia. Established gardens, kids on bicycles doing tricks over a make-shift jump made from an upturned wheel barrow and a couple of planks. Mrs Dobbinsk sitting behind a lace curtain taking notes on the comings and goings in the street. Mr Wallenstein with his German shepherd that would definitely have bitten the legs off any child who attempted to fetch the football they had just kicked over the fence. In fact, Mr Wallenstein's German shepherd was almost as frightening as Mr Wallenstein's hare lip. Then there was Niki Prowvik, who had lice. All the time. It was a typical Canberra middle class suburb.

Nigel took the entry curb a little quickly and as we bumped back down there was the most enormous BANG! The bang was followed by scraping, crunching, and ripping. In what seemed like an eternity but I imagine was really a matter of less than a second, the radio stopped and the Skoda's engine came ripping through to join us in the front seats. There was the engine, poking its head into the cabin, still running! Sitting in between us, with the radio and dashboard all bent up around it, the engine spluttered much like an old man might on a sinewy bit of lamb. Then it conked out with a last hurrah, a fizz not unlike the noise my son Henry and I make when we release the air brake on a big pretend truck. Finally a long eerie wheeze.

Then silence.

NM: "Now there is something you don't see every day Lorimer Moseley. Closest I've ever been to a car engine.

Filthy things aren't they? Do you mind walking the last bit? I don't like to draw attention to myself."

LM: *"Sure Nigel Mawson. Do you want me to call Road Service or anything?"*

NM: *"You best not. Car's not registered and I don't exist."*

Nigel got his bag out of the trunk, turned around and walked up the street, leaving the Skoda SuperSport 110 smoking away at the top of my street.

LM: *"See you Nigel Mawson."*

NM: *"See you Lorimer Moseley."*

I joined the kids in investigating it and we all agreed to pretend it had been dumped. Mrs Dobbinsk would know better but we all knew she would have to die before anyone could read her notes. When the council fellow came to take the Skoda away he couldn't believe what he saw. The bolts that held the engine to the frame of the car were missing. In fact, *everything* that held the engine to the frame was missing. The noise that Nigel was trying to avoid was in fact the engine slowly coming loose. It took a year, but eventually the whole engine just fell out and the Skoda SuperSport 110 died.

so, what does Nigel's Skoda Supersport 110 have to do with pain?

The one sentence take home message: Pain is a critical protective device – ignore it at your own peril.

I like Nigel's SuperSkoda 110 story because it shows how important it is to respect the warning signs. For Nigel, it was the noise of something going wrong under the bonnet (hood). Sure, he *could* do things to conceal the signs - to *'anaesthetise'* the noise perhaps. But in the end this was not a very sensible thing to do and the cost was, well, the cost was the SuperSport 110. Not a major cost perhaps but the point is there.

Of course, ignoring pain doesn't always lead to destruction of the painful part alone. Check out Crazy Kivin's experience.......

crazy kivin's brush with death.

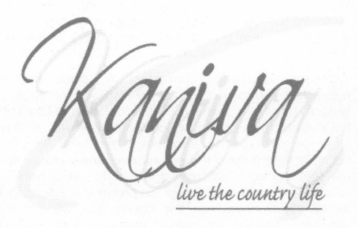

Or: Pain is what tells us to protect our body.

One of the best ways to travel around Australia is to hitchhike. Granted, it is not for everyone, but it certainly was for me. A few mates and I set up an annual hitchhiking race, whereby we would all meet for breakfast and set up a staggered start. The agreement was that when you reached the target town, you had to get your race card stamped by the barman at a pre-designated pub. It was, therefore, a time trial. Winner got all expenses reimbursed by the other racers and then gave half of it to a charity.

If the target town was far enough away, you would often run into each other along the way. Occasionally you would fly past another racer while they waited on the side of the road for a lift. We implemented a time-exchange program, whereby if you convinced your lift to stop for a competitor, the competitor was required to donate you 30 minutes in exchange for first dibs at the next point. Most trips were for a long weekend. The longest was from Sydney to a place called Kaniva, in country Victoria. 1165 km[4]. This was my best performance, and possibly the best performance by anyone hitchhiking, anywhere. Ever. It was certainly the best in the 6 year history of the Annual Hitchhiking Race for Charity[5].

As usual, we met for breakfast at Badde Manors, a reasonably grungy café on St John's Road in Glebe, inner western suburbs of Sydney. Later we shifted to Digi.Kaf, the first cyber café in town, which would end up hosting me while I wrote up my doctoral thesis. They (well, Susie really – I am not sure if Paul, the owner, ever knew about it) kept me well stocked with very good coffee and panini and soups and little treats. "All for the progress of science" Susie would say. Anyway, on the Kaniva trip, we left Badde Manors in staggered fashion between 9.40 and 11.20. There were six of us. I was last.

It was tricky, as always, to get out of Sydney. Technically, we were permitted to take a bus, but it cost 30 minutes per dollar, which is pretty expensive, so no-one really did. Trains and taxis were banned. Usually, the best plan was to head

---

4 1165 km is about 726.5 miles.
5 Team T-shirts: We thought it was funny first year of the race to call it the First Annual Hitchhiking Race for Charity, and got printed T-shirts with "FAHRC – Beat your mates to home base". Then again, we *were* 22.

down to one of the main distributors that headed out of town and to stick a sign up. A few of the boys made their first sign over breakfast and our endeavours became the talk of the café. My signs were always a bit more melodramatic than the others. For example, Dicko might write a sign like this:

```
┌─────────────────────────────┐
│ ┌─────────────────────────┐ │
│ │                         │ │
│ │        SOUTH            │ │
│ │                         │ │
│ └─────────────────────────┘ │
└─────────────────────────────┘
```

Whereas I would write a sign like this:

```
┌─────────────────────────────┐
│ ┌─────────────────────────┐ │
│ │   Heading SOUTH.        │ │
│ │   Racing my mates. I    │ │
│ │   won't sing. I PROMISE.│ │
│ └─────────────────────────┘ │
└─────────────────────────────┘
```

On the back of my signs, I always wrote a pleasant farewell, because I think everyone who *considers* stopping for a hitchhiker but *doesn't stop for them* – you know - takes their foot off the throttle a bit but goes on anyway – has a look in the rear-view mirror to confirm the wisdom of their choice. So, I wrote this on the back:

15

> # No worries. Have a
> # GREAT day!

The flipside message got me at least one lift. That was in wheat country in western NSW. A farmer reversed about 400 metres to pick me up after reading:

> # No problem. I hope it's
> # a bumper crop this
> # year!

As it turned out, the Kaniva trip didn't need a sign. I packed up our plates and took them into the kitchen, had a final chat to the cook, whose kiddies I was babysitting the following Friday, and picked up my bag. I was just about to step out and stroll down to the eastern distributor when a fellow on the opposite side of the café remarked:

"Did I hear thet you are going to Kaniva?"

I responded in the affirmative and then got a barrage of questions:

"Why?

LM: "Hitchhiking race"

"Why?"

LM: "Fun, primarily, and we raise money for MissionBeat or Salvo's or someone like that"

"Kun yer talk?"

LM: "Yes"

"Are yer posh?"

LM: "I don't reckon. What do you reckon Cook? Am I posh?"

Cook: "About as posh as my Rottweiler"

"Kun yer drive?"

LM: "Yes"

"I'll take yer thun"

LM (a little uncomfortable): "Sorry?"

"I'll take yer thun. Kaniva. I'm huddin to Lullumur. Nuxt town along. Be good to huv company. Uvin uf you are un Aussie."

So there it was. A lift. From start to finish. And that is how I met Crazy Kivin. Kevin was his real name but he was a Kiwi and I can't help talking like a Kiwi whenever I spend time with Kiwi's (you may have picked this up already). Crazy Kiv drove a reasonably old Mazda ute[6]. Two seats, flat tray. He was parked (illegally) right at the front door of Badde Manors. We got in and started chatting. He was a most intriguing fellow. He was heading to Lillimur to meet a Bull Mastif that he was thinking about buying. His ute was small and the engine worked hard, especially when we got out of Sydney into the glorious southern tablelands.

---

6 Ute: Ute is short for utility – a bit like a pick-up truck only smaller.

Farmers have them mostly. Crazy's ute looked a bit like this:

Crazy and I rattled past the Dog on the Tuckerbox just outside of Gundagai, and turned off the main drag, onto the Sturt Highway and towards Wagga Wagga. That was about 5 hours in. The ute was low on fuel so we stopped in at Wagga[7], which is when Crazy asked me to drive.

We were not back on the highway for more than a few minutes when the exclamation mark light came on. I have always loved the exclamation mark light. It is completely uninformative except to say *"something* is wrong *somewhere,* but I'm not going to tell you exactly *where"*. Crazy's ute was manufactured when cars were just getting fitted with little computers that would tell you stuff about the car. More information than the usual temperature, oil and brake lights on the dash. The computers were sophisticated enough to tell you something was wrong, but you had to find out yourself what exactly it was (bit like psychotherapy I guess). I mentioned the recently illuminated light to Crazy –

> *LM: "Hey Kiv – we better check thus out – your warning light is on"*
>
> *Crazy Kevin: "Yeah I know hey bro'. It comes on a but – bin on sunce before Gundagai. Doesn't seem to be a problem though ey?"*
>
> *LM: "It might be Kiv. Why don't you take a look in the manual, see what utt says?"*
>
> *CK: "Naah. It'll be alright bro'"*

He seemed to not worry at all about it, but it did concern me. I had driven my girlfriend's dad's car for a few minutes after the exclamation mark light came on and ended up

---

7 Wagga Wagga: It is only permissible to call Wagga Wagga 'Wagga', if you have spent enough time in Wagga Wagga to realise that Wagga Wagga is not 'Wagga', but that 'Wagga' is an affectionate shortening of Wagga Wagga. Otherwise, always call Wagga Wagga Wagga Wagga.

with a cracked head gasket (on the car, not on me). So, I was pretty insistent with Kiv. He cracked.

CK: "Alright yer bug worry wart. You keep drivung and I wull fux utt up."

With that, Crazy got something from under his seat and then leaned over towards me. He stuck his head up under the dash. He was fiddling around there for a while (this made me a little uncomfortable), and then with a final click, something happened and the light went off. He came out with a little globe in his hand.

CK: "There utt is. No worries now. Won't bother you a but."

This was indeed a novel strategy and one that didn't sit too comfortably with me. I drove on and, funnily enough, forgot about it. That is until we passed the turn off into Narrandera, at which point we headed south toward Deniliquin and the Mallee country. This time a big P illuminated on the left of the dash, just above where the exclamation mark had been.

LM: "Hey Kiv, what does P mean, on the dash?"

CK: "Stuffed uf I know bro'. Panic? Ho ho fruggin ho?"

LM: "Thunk we should stop Kiv? Take a look under the bonnet perhaps?"

CK: "Naah – I'll fux utt up – I know cars"

Again he leaned over and fiddled behind the dash, emerging with another little globe and a look of satisfaction. The most amazing thing was how easily I tended to forget about the two little lights. We went another hundred miles or so when a third light came on. This one looked like a water jug. Again, Crazy just leaned over and emerged a few minutes later with the globe. He was positively chuffed with his little haul of globes and began tossing them back and forth in his hands. The thing was, I began to think that this was truly avoiding the problem – the ute was running well, it didn't *seem* sick in any way, and Kiv seemed to know *exactly* what he was doing. The last light to come on had a picture of what looked vaguely like a foot on a brake pedal. I told Kiv and this time he lent right across me and pulled a fuse out of the little black box near my knee. All the dash lights went out.

> CK: *"Sorted hey Bro'. Now you won't get* any *lights tellung you* anything *now."*

Sure enough, we rolled into the Commercial Hotel in Kaniva at 11.46. We were just in time for last drinks and the barman signed my card: "23:52 Friday." It had taken me 12 hours and 52 minutes to travel 1165 kilometres. That is unbelievable hitchhiking time.

After closing, Crazy set up the swag[8] on the back of the ute and I slept under the tray. The sun came up about a millisecond before the council street cleaner sprayed me with water. We were both up and Crazy got in the ute so he could see this Bull Mastiff first thing – his theory was that dogs are always grumpy before breakfast, so before breakfast was the only time to tell for sure if it was a "Heckyl

---

8 A swag: A swag is a roll-up canvas bed, complete with mattress and bedding.

20

or a Jive[9] – makes all the difference". I bid him farewell and he took off up the main street.

I have this thing about watching people as they drive off. I have to watch them until they are out of sight. I think it is a legacy of standing on the street as a kid waving my grandparents off as they headed back home after a couple of weeks with our family. Nanna would have her arm out waving the whole time and we would all wave as long as we could see them and then turn around and notice Mum's tears, not really knowing what to do about them. Crazy was no more than a couple of hundred yards away when his left indicator came on but I could hear the ute accelerating into the corner. In fact, it didn't turn the corner at all. Instead it just accelerated straight across the road, jumped the kerb and blew up. It turned into a speeding fire ball, still accelerating, careering across a big carpark until it met with a brick fence at which time it stopped dead still, on fire, back wheels spinning madly in thin air.

Crazy Kivin dropped out onto the ground and crawled away. By the time I got to him he looked bad. There was a whole lot of blood. He already had a lump the size of a golf ball on the left side of his forehead and a gash across his cheek. He explained that the steering and brakes went and the car just started accelerating. Nothing he could do.

CK: *"I hope that guy from the Kaniva Times got a shot of the old girl blowing up. That'd be my 12 minutes. But you know the worst thing?"*

LM: *"What Kiv? What's the worst thing?"*

CK: *"I'll not know if that Bull Mastif is a Heckyl or a bloody Jive."*

---

9 Heckyl & Jive: Crazy's phrasing, not mine.

so, what does Crazy Kivin's brush with death have to do with pain?

The one sentence take home message: Pain is a critical protective device – ignore it at your own peril.

If Nigel attempted to *'anaesthetise'* the problem with his SuperSkoda, then Crazy Kivin might have been taking some more drastic measures. The whole point of warning lights on the dash of a car is to tell you, the driver, that something requires action. Sure, you can do things to turn the light off – to *anaesthetise* the dash perhaps. To *surgically remove* the apparent culprit, or end up doing *neurolysis*[10] on the whole electric supply, but if your clinical reasoning is not sound, then there might be a major cost. The cost for Kevin was not simply that part of his ute that was in danger. Rather, the cost for Kevin was (almost) *everything*. Death. Kaput. All over. Both Crazy Kivin and Nigel were attempting to remove pain, rather than remove the cause(s) of pain. In Nigel's case, it was a specific pathology (problem) with the engine's attachment to the car. In Kivin's case, there were many contributing factors and he just kept removing his ute's ability to tell the driver about it.

It is clear that both Nigel and Kivin were spectacularly stupid people. If they ever read this I imagine they will think the whole thing is a tribute to their cleverness. That is another amazing thing - Kivin convinced me that what he was doing was *not stupid*. Simply by knowing a whole lot about cars, or at least seeming to, I figured there was no reason to doubt him.

---

10 Neurolysis: Neurolysis refers to the destruction of nerves, or nerve tissue, by burning it, cutting it, or injecting it with chemicals.

I think there are plenty of things about these stories that make them useful metaphors for patients in pain. They remind us that pain is a warning system, which usually gives us early warning of something in the body going, or about to go, awry. To devise strategies that effectively remove that system is, ultimately, going to be problematic. In this sense, I have told this story to patients with the following types of issues:

1. Athletes who push their bodies so hard that the normal pain protective system doesn't work very well. If patients don't change their behaviour in response to pain, then pain hasn't achieved its goal.

2. Patients who don't care what is wrong with them as long as they can find someone to 'block it again', or a drug that will turn it off, so that they can go back to their full lifestyle straight away without having to actively do anything to help themselves (in a rehabilitation sense).

3. Patients who are keen to use TENS or drugs as their main pain management strategy. This scenario is similar to (2) but also slightly different. For the TENS thing, I find patients are really receptive to Nigel's SuperSport 110 story because of the whole turn the radio up so that the *fuzzy* noise is louder than the noise coming from the problem – it is an obvious link to the proposed mechanisms of TENS – to use non-noxious[11] input to inhibit the noxious input.

4. Those patients who tend to avoid things because they know that they will hurt. I use Crazy Kivin's strategy of simply removing the light globes that lit up the various lights as a metaphor of the way some patients tend to avoid the pain, but don't address the underlying problem.

---

11 Noxious means dangerous. Think of noxious chemicals, noxious weeds – they are dangerous chemicals and dangerous weeds. A nociceptor is a special type of nerve that responds to anything that is dangerous. For example, dangerously hot, dangerously cold, dangerously low on oxygen, dangerously high in acid. We have nociceptors in almost every tissue in our body.

seeing is believing

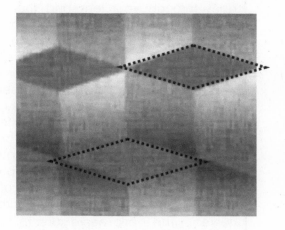

Or, pain doesn't provide a measure of the state
of the tissues.

I remember quite clearly being told about how visual
perception works. I was sitting up the back of Mrs Smart's
Social Psychology class at Hawker College. I chose social
psychology as an elective because my brother did. For

some reason I had come to expect that doing psychology would make me a better person, or it would at least increase my chances of developing deeply rewarding relationships in the future. There was, after-all, no higher calling than 'to relate' (jeepers I took some things too seriously – while I was learning social psychology my mates were doing experiments with grasshoppers and planning how to pash Suzanne Jackson behind the tennis wall). I think my mum had been able to convince me that I was naturally good at psych-type things so I figured that doing it at school would get me a few easy marks. The first unit, Visual Perception 101, was pretty easy. According to Mrs Smart, visual perception works like this:

> If you point your eye in the direction of something, the light that is reflected from that thing enters your eye, goes through your lens and then hits your retina. Upside-down. Everyone always remembers that – as though it is one of the most remarkable things in the entire animal kingdom. I reckon it shows how boring the rest of it must have been. Your retina consists of millions of cells that are super-duper light receptors. Different types of light receptors are activated by light of different wavelengths (it is the different frequencies that we end up seeing as different colours – actually I think colour depends on the *relationship* between the light energy and its wavelength – but all that is a bit beside the point here). Activation of these receptors causes action potentials in the neurons of your optic nerve[12]. The optic nerve runs to the *primary visual cortex*, which is in your occipital lobe. The primary visual cortex consists of 20 million neurons, which flip the image back the right way so that you get a conscious experience of the light that is entering your eye.

---

12 Nerve or tract?: Technically, the optic nerve is a tract, not a nerve. Tracts don't leave the central nervous system, whereas nerves do.

This, apparently, was vision. I learnt later, in physiotherapy school, that there are cones and rods and a fovum and the yadda yadda yadda layer[13]. Despite this substantial leap in knowledge of the visual system, the principle seemed the same and that is: the visual system is a very specific and reliable system so that what you see is what you get – you see a direct representation of what is entering your eye.

I am not sure that Mrs Smart's Social Psychology class lived up to my expectations. Not all was lost though - my mates didn't gain too much from their grasshopper experiments, nor from Suzanne Jackson I imagine. One thing that Mrs Smart did leave with me however, was a restless whispering in the back of my mind, that surely it can't be that simple. Here are three questions I asked Mrs Smart:

1. Do we really need 20 million neurones in the visual cortex just to flip an image?

2. How do I see things in my sleep if my eyes are closed?

3. How do visual illusions work?

This is how the conversation went:

> LM: *"That seems a rather large number of neurons and a large amount of space, just to flip the image back the other way. Why don't we just have another retina there and use the spare neurones and brain space to think with?"*

---

13 The yadda yadda yadda layer: This is not the real name of the layer of photosensitive neuronal cells that sit underneath the cones and rods that make up the retina, but it will do.

Mrs Smart: "Lorimer my boy, we are indeed fearfully and wonderfully made."

LM: "What sort of a ridiculous answer is that!"

I didn't actually say the last bit because Social Psychology had taught me that to do so would not be conducive to mutually respectful interaction. However, I did think it and I reckon I may have even mouthed the "Wha-" before regaining an attitude of mutual respect over my motor output.

This interaction dealt my naturally inquisitive nature a steady blow. Up until then Mrs Smart had been right up there with Mary Poppins and Carla (Captain Kremmen's wonderful assistant on the 'Kenny Everett Video Show') as truly unfaultable women. But "we are indeed fearfully and wonderfully made" really got me. I had all these insulting lines running through my head: "Smart is obviously not your maiden name" etc etc. Even though I was not the sort of fellow who would normally express myself in that way, it was probably only my substantial crush on Mrs Smart's daughter Naomi, that stopped me.

So, the whisperings in my mind stayed with me, right up to physiotherapy school. I was so excited about Perception with Professor Ron Balnar, that I arrived for the first lesson pretty much on time. It is the only time I can remember that I was first to class. I liked Prof Balnar – he had this peculiar habit of taking a very large stick with him wherever he went. He would start each lecture with something like:

"Mmm, my stick, large isn't it? Anyway, it won't be going anywhere. Was tree just weeks ago I'm dashed – such is the way though. Such is the way. Tree to stick. Matter of connection. And context I guess. Now there's a thought...."

Like most nutty professors, he seemed to be terrifically clever and terrifically stupid at the same time. I was sure that his knowledge of vision would calm my disquiet. I waited with bated breath for him to answer my three questions as he took us on a tour of the human nervous system. He doddered on until I lost patience and asked him directly:

> *LM: "That seems a rather large number of neurons and a large amount of space, just to flip the image back the other way. Why don't we just have another retina there?"*
>
> *Prof Balnar: "Yes, yes it does doesn't it. Yes. Good point. Quite so. Would a retina work there? Mmm. Would it. Not sure. Good point. Good question. Might evolution have missed that? Not all luck of course. Where is my stick?"*

So. Prof Balnar was about as helpful as Mrs Smart. As it turns out, Mrs Smart's position on it has proved more useful for me than Prof Balnar's – every time my neuroscience journal contents email alert pops into my inbox, I become more convinced that we are indeed fearfully and wonderfully constructed. Mrs Smart has become the new whispering in my head.

I headed into the textbooks. It seems that there is a great deal more going on when we see. This is some of what I learnt:

Light does in fact reflect off your environment and land on your retina and it does in fact invert on its way through your eyeball, which means it does land on your retina upside down (thank God for that – what would we have done if we leant that *that* was a bumsteer?!). Light does in fact stimulate cones and rods on your retina and it does in fact send that information through your optic nerves to the back of your brain – your occipital cortex. That is where the story becomes fundamentally different. A most magnificent thing happens: instantaneously and *without you knowing*, your brain calls on all sorts of previous experiences: the things you have learnt - things that you know that you know and things that you don't know that you know, your expectations, other sensory inputs, explicit memories and implicit memories.

All of those things can activate neurones in the brain, which in turn can mould and massage, modify and modulate the information that has been sent from the retina. The *conscious* experience of vision emerges *after* this highly sophisticated modulation process. There is no doubt that light hitting your retina is very very important, but light is neither sufficient nor necessary for you to have a visual experience. Proof of the former is found in visual illusions, when you see things that are not there. Proof of the latter is found when you dream and your eyes are closed. That points to what I reckon is a really important thing - your brain *creates* your visual experience. That visual experience is not simply a picture of what is entering your eye, it is an interpretation of that information.

What we see, then is not *'the facts'*, but a sensible image, based on the original light information, but modulated, perhaps tailor-made, for you[14].

Take for example, figure 1. Do the lines look the same length? Even if you have seen this before and you *know* that they are the same length, they probably *look* different.

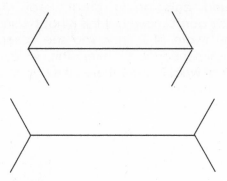

Figure 1 Lines of the same length look different

Try looking at this picture for just a split second – a backwards blink if you like. Notice that they still look different! Try looking at it for a while and try to make the lines look the same length – you can probably feel that you are trying to block out certain bits of information in the picture. You might have some luck by making your eyes go sufficiently blurry so as to make the lines almost impossible to detect. But then the picture is completely meaningless.

Taking into consideration things that you know (but you don't know that you know) is not just about geometry. Have a look at the image in figure 2. In this figure, square A is definitely darker than square B right? Wrong.

---

14 Seeing is interpretation: The indefatigable Chris Murphy told me that this reminded him of a saying in NLP: "the map is not the territory", which Smurphy reckons means that what you see is not what is really there, but your interpretation.

If you don't believe this, grab a piece of paper and cut out holes for the panels. So, what is going on there? Lots, apparently. The caption quotes the inventor of this illusion in his explanation. If you are interested, take a look at his chapter on this type of thing in the reference list Ref List No. 2.

If you are like me, you might be satisfied with a fairly broad explanation like this: in a split second, and outside of your consciousness, your brain processes a great deal of information and calls on a great deal of previous knowledge. You don't know that this is happening. The first thing you are aware of is. that you see a sensible and meaningful 3-dimensional picture. This is a conscious representation of what is really there. It is not accurate, but it is meaningful and sensible.

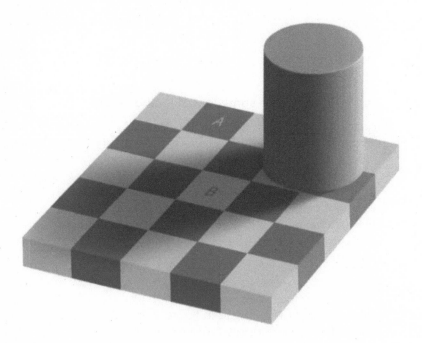

Figure 2 The same colour illusion

This illusion, and the one at the front of this chapter, in which the two diamonds are really the same shade of grey, shows the way the brain can modulate light information so that it makes sense, rather than give you a truly accurate conscious experience of what is hitting your retina. This one is called the same colour illusion, published by Ted Adelson in 1995 (it is sometimes called Adelson's checker shadow illusion). Although squares A and B are the same shade of grey, square A appears darker. I got Ted Adelson's own explanation from his website (he said I could stick it in my book). This is the website:

http://web.mit.edu/persci/people/adelson/checkershado wdescription.html

This is the explanation:

> *The visual system needs to determine the color of objects in the world. In this case the problem is to determine the gray shade of the checks on the floor. Just measuring the light coming from a surface (the luminance) is not enough: a cast shadow will dim a surface, so that a white surface in shadow may be reflecting less light than a black surface in full light. The visual system uses several tricks to determine where the shadows are and how to compensate for them, in order to determine the shade of gray "paint" that belongs to the surface. The first trick is based on local contrast. In shadow or not, a check that is lighter than its neighboring checks is probably lighter than average, and vice versa. In the figure, the light check in shadow is surrounded by darker checks. Thus, even though the check is physically dark, it is light when compared to its neighbors. The dark checks outside the shadow, conversely, are surrounded by lighter checks, so they look dark by comparison. A second trick is based on the fact that shadows often have soft edges, while paint boundaries (like the checks) often have sharp edges. The visual system tends to ignore gradual changes in light level, so that it can determine the color of the surfaces without being misled by shadows. In this figure, the shadow looks like a shadow, both because it is fuzzy and because the*

33

shadow casting object is visible. The "paintness" of the checks is aided by the form of the "X-junctions" formed by 4 abutting checks. This type of junction is usually a signal that all the edges should be interpreted as changes in surface color rather than in terms of shadows or lighting. As with many so-called illusions, this effect really demonstrates the success rather than the failure of the visual system.

The visual system is not very good at being a physical light meter, but that is not its purpose. The important task is to break the image information down into meaningful components, and thereby perceive the nature of the objects in view.

It was me, not Ted, who made that bold. I did so because it is a beautiful conclusion and one that is so immediately applicable to pain. Watch this:

The ~~visual~~ PAIN system is not very good at being a physical ~~light~~ DAMAGE meter, but that is not its purpose. The important task is to break the ~~image~~ information down into meaningful components, and thereby perceive the ~~nature of the objects in view~~ NEED FOR ACTION.

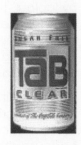

The spectacular flop of clear cola

This modulation of sensory input is not unique to vision. The worldwide flop of Clear Cola (Tab Clear© was Coca-Cola©'s particular version) demonstrated that taste is just as open to modulation as vision is. Clear colas were clear, like lemonade, but clear cola tasted like normal cola. Actually, clear cola tasted like normal cola if you couldn't see it, but it didn't if you could. This meant that people would drink clear cola if it came out of a can because it tasted just like normal cola that way. But they wouldn't drink it if it came out of a bottle or a glass, because it didn't taste like real cola then. Let's face it, if you drink clear cola from a can, no one else can see how groovy you are because you're drinking cola that is clear. What then, is the point? You might as well drink normal cola. So the whole thing flopped – the end of clear cola. And the creative team that thought of it I bet. Good work guys.

The point is this: that clear cola was no good when you could see it shows that the brain uses visual information to mould, modify and modulate the sensory information coming from the taste buds. When you see that it looks like lemonade, the conscious experience that emerges is, it seems, not that good. Considering that normal cola is bad enough, it strikes me that clear cola may well have been very rank indeed. Still, it seems that there may be a few odd bods that are still fans of the clear stuff. Tab Clear hasn't been made for more than a decade, but I just put £17.21 on an unopened bottle on E-bay...and got outbid!

An alternative way to experience the modulation of taste by colour is by doing the following experiment. I have found it useful for convincing patients about the way the brain messes with sensory information, but it is most entertaining if you do it with your kids (or, if you don't have any kids, borrow someone else's).

Get some lime soda. Pour two glasses of it and in one glass put some green food colouring. Ask the kiddies which drink has the more intense flavour (don't tell them it is a trick because they will tell you the opposite of what they really think because they want to out-trick you! Actually, I might do that.)

This type of experiment has been undertaken in proper controlled environments by real-life scientists. In a range of studies, colour and viscosity have been shown to affect different aspects of taste and smell (e.g. sweetness, intensity, presumed calorie content, odour). The magnitude of the effect seems to relate to the age of the subject, which means that the older you get, the more you learn and the more your brain gets tricked by such things [Ref List No. 3].

so what has all that got to do with pain?

The one sentence take home message: Pain, like vision, is a conscious experience that is based on many complex processes, not just the sensory information coming from your body (or, for vision, eyes).

There are several things about vision that I think are particularly useful for understanding pain. More to the point,

36

there are several *principles* of vision that can be applied to pain and help us to see that the brain is a very clever thing indeed. Here are what I consider to be the key points:

1. Vision seems simple. More simple than pain at least. However, even vision is dependent on complex evaluative processes. What you see is not what you get, but rather the end result of many inputs. The conscious experience is based·on all you know, what you know you know but more so on what you don't know that you know. Because the brain is able to do this, what we *actually see* is sensible, and therefore biologically advantageous.

    Pain is like this too – *the brain evaluates the sensory input from the tissues of the body and draws on complex evaluative processes. Pain then, can be considered a conscious experience based on the brain's evaluation of how much danger the tissues are in.*

2. Evaluation of all the other stuff happens *really* quickly and outside of your awareness and control. No one would expect you to consciously decide what to see on the basis of previous experience, calculating light vectors (in your head as you go!), blurred edges etc. No one would imply that you are seeing an illusion because you are consciously deciding to see an illusion and that you are just after some attention or someone to compensate you for seeing that illusion.

    Pain is like this too – *the evaluation of how much danger the tissues are actually in happens really quickly and outside of your awareness and control. Pain then, depends on the unconscious evaluation of threat to body tissue.*

37

the thirsty idiots

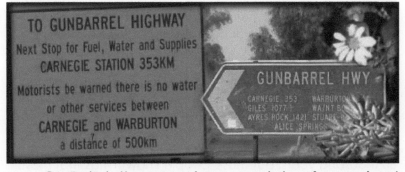

TO GUNBARREL HIGHWAY
Next Stop for Fuel, Water and Supplies
CARNEGIE STATION 353KM
Motorists be warned there is no water
or other services between
CARNEGIE and WARBURTON
a distance of 500km

GUNBARREL HWY
CARNEGIE 353   WARBURTO
GILES 1077   WAJNT BO
AYRES ROCK 1421 STUAR
ALICE SPRING

Or: Pain is the conscious correlate of perceived threat to tissues that motivates us to get our tissues out of danger.

There's a road in Australia called the Gunbarrel Highway. It might be a bit generous to call it a road – in some places it has not been graded since it was originally constructed, several decades ago. It is about 1400 km long. It is called the Gunbarrel Highway because the lead surveyor had a thing for neat straight lines on maps, so he did his best to make the highway as straight as possible. Because of the long straight stretches, his construction team got the nickname the 'gunbarrel team' and the name stuck. The highway links Wiluna in the west with Giles in the east. Wiluna is about 500 km nor-noreast of Kalgoorlie. Kalgoorlie is about 600 km east of Perth. Perth is officially the most isolated city in the world. I don't know what that makes Wiluna, but it sure doesn't have a Tube station. Giles is not far from Uluru[15], that mighty monolith right at the heart of the Australian continent and its people.

Why one might want to link Wiluna and Giles is not completely obvious. Wiluna consists of a service station, to service vehicles as they prepare for, or recover from, the Highway; a general store; a pub and a camping ground. Giles consists of a remote meteorology station, known as Giles. The initial reason for building the road was to service a weapons research facility called Woomera. This part of Australia was considered by the British to be the best place in the world for a rocket range, presumably because it was a long way from Britain, and from where British constituents lived. It is certainly a part of the world not well suited to Europeans or their frigid descendents. Of course, people have been living happily in that part of the world for about 60 thousand years, but those people know things that most of us don't. At each end of the Gunbarrel Highway, there are strong warnings to take sufficient water for two days and enough fuel to get between stops, the longest gap being 600 km.

One pair of clever fellows, Adam and Tony, decided to drive the Gunbarrel Highway in their Lada Niva, as fast as they could. They were, apparently, experienced outback adventurers. They were also New Zealanders, which casts some doubt over the 'outbackness' of their adventuring, but that is a bit by the by. Adam and Tony had well designated roles and followed all the normal procedures.

---

15 Uluru: Once known as Ayers Rock

That didn't make up for the fact that they were in a Lada Niva, a vehicle notorious for being crap. The Lada lived up to its reputation and broke down smack bang in the middle of the longest unbroken stretch on the highway. All the electronics were out, which meant the car wouldn't work. More importantly, it meant the two-way radio wouldn't work.

These two fellows – Adam and Tony, were a thousand kilometres from anywhere worth being. It would have been 55°C in the shade (~ 130°F), if there was any shade. The point is, it was hot. Damn hot. This is obviously a potentially dangerous situation. Any experienced rally team would be prepared for such an event and indeed, Adam and Tony were prepared, although they didn't realise it.

One designated role that Adam had was to pack the water. After an hour or so in desert sun he went to get the water out of the back of the Lada and saw that it was missing. Adam told Tony that somehow he must have forgotten to pack the water. They resigned themselves to having to sit it out – the ranger at Giles would expect them in about two days time and would give them a few hours grace. Adam and Tony hoped that help would arrive before death did and if not, that death would arrive via sleep and not via the dingo's and eagles that would already be aware of the lame kiwis lying underneath their Lada Niva.

Now in this situation, one is sweating, as they say, 'like a pig' (which is a daft saying because pigs don't sweat). Sweating leads to dehydration, which makes one thirsty. We all know that thirst is pretty much an upside down measure of hydration (or a right-way up measure of dehydration). Don't we? Read on my fellow hydroheathens! As time went on, these two lads were getting very, very dehydrated. They were also getting very, very thirsty. Just less than 48 hours later, they heard the distinctive drizzly drone of the Royal Flying Doctor Service Cessna and scrambled, with what little energy they had, to get something to wave. There on the back seat was a silver thermal blanket, which would contrast beautifully with the red sands of the desert. On ripping the blanket out, Tony saw, and immediately remembered, that when he replaced the spare wheel, he had moved the water from the trunk to underneath the thermal blanket on the back seat. They were so thirsty that the sight of the water sent them into a frenzy. They waved the sheet, noted the change in trajectory of the Cessna, which indicated that they had been seen, and started drinking. Adam and Tony drank like they were on their last legs, which they were.

Here is the groovy bit – by guzzling down a couple of litres or so of water, their thirst was quenched. The plane landed, the paramedics arrived, Adam and Tony indicated that *they were not thirsty* because they had just had plenty of water to drink. In actual fact, they were still so dangerously dehydrated that both lost consciousness before the plane had swung around to head for Kalgoorlie Base Hospital.

Aside from narrowly missing the Darwin Awards[16], Adam and Tony's experience demonstrates a critical aspect of thirst. After their big drink they were then *no longer thirsty*, but they were still *severely dehydrated*. So, thirst does not tell us about hydration. Rather, it makes us drink. It works like this:

> *As you become dehydrated, blood volume starts to drop and receptors in your cardiovascular system respond to that drop. These receptors sit on the end of small diameter myelinated neurons. When the receptors are activated, they cause those neurones to send action potentials into the central nervous system and thence to the brain. The brain, outside of consciousness, evaluates this information in light of every other piece of*

---

16 The Darwin Awards: The Darwin Awards are given to people who die because they did a remarkably stupid thing. The awards honour the contribution that such morons make to natural selection, by removing themselves from the gene pool. http://www.darwinawards.com/

information available, and evokes a response. In the first instance, the response may be to constrict blood vessels, reduce blood flow to non-critical areas, reduce respiratory rate. If the brain evaluates the situation as requiring a behavioural response from the organism, *then a conscious experience will emerge – thirst. That's the thing about thirst – it is the single best way to get someone to drink. As the proverb goes – 'You can take a horse to water but you can't make it drink. Unless it is thirsty.'*[17] *So, it is thirst that motivates us to do what is required to get a drink. When you look at it this way, it is clear to see that thirst is a conscious experience that makes us do something. The Wiggles, a children's music band and Australia's most successful entertainers, put it so eloquently in their* absolute *classic: "Drink drink, drink some water, it's so good for you."*

The other critical thing about this system is that when the brain is satisfied that enough has been done, then it will stop creating the experience of thirst. This is how we can make sense of what happened to Adam and Tony.

so, what have the thirsty idiots got to do with pain?

The one sentence take home message: Pain, like thirst, is a conscious experience that *motivates* you to do something to protect your body.

---

17 Dodgy proverb: This may not be a completely accurate account of the famous proverb.

These are the points that I like to get out of this story:

1. Thirst, like vision, is an experience we are all pretty comfortable with, not stigmatised, and so-on and so-forth. Thirst, like vision (and pain), is dependent on unconscious evaluative brain processes, such that it does not accurately reflect the world, but our place in it.

2. Thirst is a conscious experience that motivates us to do something to survive. The reason that it is effective is that it is sufficiently unpleasant to make us want to stop it. That is, **thirst does not provide a measure of dehydration, thirst makes us drink.**

    *Pain is like this. Pain is a conscious experience that motivates us to do something to protect the tissues that the brain perceives to be under threat. Explain Pain [Ref List No. 1] and Patrick Wall's superb book, Pain: The science of suffering [Ref List No. 4] make this point really clear, by drawing on experimental and anecdotal evidence. That is, **pain does not provide a measure of the state of the tissues, pain makes us do something to protect tissues that are perceived to be under threat.***

3. When the brain is satisfied that enough has been done, it will stop *creating* the experience of thirst. This confirms that thirst is not a measure of hydration. If it was, Tony and Adam would have been thirsty until their hydration was back to normal. I reckon that the 25 minutes or so between drinking the water and blood volume etc returning to normal is the most poignant aspect of the story because there was severe dehydration and no thirst. This proves that thirst is not a measure of hydration.

    Pain is like this. If the brain is satisfied that enough has been done to get the tissues out of danger, then it stops making the body part painful. This is a really nice way of understanding why inert pills and injections can still reduce pain – the brain has every good reason to conclude that what you have just done should reduce the danger level, so it reduces the pain. There are good studies that look at how it does this and we know it involves opiate-related and non-opiate related bits[18]. If you take this principle further, you can say that if pain reduces, it shows that the perceived threat to body tissues has reduced. It is very tricky to know what it was that changed that perception. This principle is defended in the following papers and chapters:

1. *Melzack, R. Gate control theory. On the evolution of pain concepts. Pain Forum 5, 128-38 (1996).*

2. *Wall, P. in Ciba foundation symposium 174, experimental and theoretical studies of consciousness 187-216 (Wiley, New York, 1993).*

3. *Wall, P. Pain. The science of suffering (Orion Publishing, London, 1999).*

4. *Moseley, G. L. A pain neuromatrix approach to patients with chronic pain. Man Ther 8, 130-140 (2003).*

5. *Moseley, G. L. Reconceptualising pain according to its underlying biology. Physical Therapy Reviews. In Press (2007).*

6. *Jones, L. & Moseley, G. L. in Tidy's physiotherapy (ed. Porter, S.) In press (Elsevier, Oxford, 2007).*

4. Thirst is not the only thing that happens when hydration reduces. Lots of things happen outside of consciousness. For example, changes in blood flow, respiration, motor output, renal flow etc. All of that

---

18 Opiate-related: Opiates are officially called *narcotic alkaloids*, which is why we call them opiates. Morphine is the most famous opiate. The opiate-related system refers to neurones that use opiates to communicate. The nervous system uses opiate-systems as natural pain-killers, but there are other pain-killing systems that don't use opiates. We call those systems non-opiate systems.

happens outside of consciousness. Thirst is a sign that the brain perceives that those things alone are not enough to maintain sufficient hydration.

Pain is like this. *When tissues are perceived to be under threat, a whole lot of stuff happens outside of your consciousness. For example, blood flow changes, motor output changes, immune system activates, autonomic system activates. Pain is a sign that the brain perceives that those things alone are not enough.*

Twonames & the magic button.

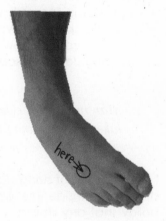

Or: The brain uses the virtual body to tell you *where* your actual body is in danger.

When you are hitch-hiking, getting out of a capital city is usually a breeze. Unless the capital city is Adelaide, in which case it is almost impossible. My average wait getting out of Adelaide is about three hours. On this occasion, it was a little over six hours since my brother had dropped me off and done his best to wish me well. He was in no state to wish me well, being rather suffocated by an irrational conviction that I was bound for death. He had told me that hitch-hikers were being organ-napped. He reckoned I would end up with my liver in Prince Myanmat of Burma and my pancreas in the son of a Vietnamese rubber mogul.

Six hours after his farewell, my rock-juggling was disrupted by the sound of a reversing car. I could tell it was reversing because it had that strained whirring noise that cars get when they reverse. The back end of a Toyota Corona was coming down the dirt strip that separated the two lanes of the highway. It zig-zagged through the dust as though it was smelling its way, like a beagle might. It dragged along a cloud of dust that looked like a sandy plumage. When the car was in line with where I stood, it stopped abruptly with a little skid and was immediately swallowed by the dustcloud. From somewhere inside the dustcloud came a vaguely frightening voice:

Man inside dust cloud: "Hey hitch-hiker, Hey Mr hitch-hiker, do yer wanna lift north? Do yer?"

I had no way of sizing up my potential lift because he was still hidden inside the cloud of dust. However, I have a policy that any lift is a good lift so I grabbed my pack, my clarinet and my hat and I ran across the road to join him. When the dust settled a fraction, I found the door, threw in my gear and jumped in the front seat. The driver of the car introduced himself:

Driver: "Simon Jeffery or Jeffery Simon — can't remember which. Been a long time since anyone knew. Got an Aunty Grace Simon 'n' an Uncle Bill Jeffery so

I'm nip the wiser. Most people call me Twonames. Want some apple?"

LM: "G'day Twonames. Lorimer. Sure"

Twonames freaked me out. Twice. First time was when he was cutting up the apple with a fishing knife that was as long as my foot and well capable, I imagined, of skinning more than just a fish. He offered me the half of the apple that was pierced atop his awfully big knife and then, as soon as I plucked the apple off the top, Twonames stabbed himself in the top of his knee. The knife made a deep thudding noise as it entered his flesh and then it just sat there, about two centimetres in, just at the top of his knee-cap, where the big leg muscles come together in a big tendon. The knife wobbled back and forth like a javelin for a second or so. I was seriously spooked. Here was this guy, in charge of a vehicle that was about take me into the South Australian outback; straight through Snowtown, a village made famous by the Snowtown murders[19]; beyond the coverage of the telephone network. A guy who has reversed his car a hundred metres to pick me up and has now stabbed himself, voluntarily, in his own leg with little more than a wimper?!?! Curiously there was no blood coming from the wound. He looked up at the knife, then at me, apple juice dripping down his chin.

Twonames: "Still gets me, that. Dunnit 50 times since the Royal and it still makes me wince. Crazy as a dog eatin' peanut butter. Every time. You better take care of this cause it just gets in me way."

---

19 Clever crimes? In the Snowtown murders, victims were killed for their social security payments and the bodies were put in a disused bank vault. It seems bizarre to me that one would take the risks involved in multiple murder, risks that I imagine are substantial, in order to collect the social security payments of the people you have murdered. If murder is your preferred means of income, would it not be more sensible to murder one rich person than a dozen poor people?

With that, Twonames lifted up his shorts and unclipped a couple of suspenders that were holding his *prosthetic* leg onto his thigh. He yanked the prosthesis off and threw it onto my lap. The thing I was to take care of was his artificial leg. Then he laughed. Well, cackled really:

> *Twonames: "You thought I'd stabbed meself didn't yer?"*
>
> *LM: "Well, yes I did Twonames. You got me with that one."*
>
> *Twonames: "Hook line and friggin' sinker I would say Warren."*
>
> *LM: "Lorimer."*
>
> *Twonames: "Borrow one? What for?"*
>
> *LM:* (it was about now I realised that Twonames' hearing loss was about the same as his leg loss) *"No no, I don't want to borrow one - my name's Lorimer."*
>
> *Twonames: "I know I know. You introduced yourself when you got in Warren."*

I left it at that. Twonames was probably pushing 50. He had a bad hair-piece, a gaunt face and sunken eyes. His skin was thin. Veins across his thighs looked like river deltas. He smelt like a pub on Sunday morning just after the Glen20[20] has been sprayed in the toilets. We took off with a jolt. Twonames explained that he had just been at the Royal Adelaide Hospital to have his stump revised[21], but had discharged himself because they wouldn't let him

---

20 Glen20: A disinfectant spray that is meant to hide smells but really just marries them.

21 Revised stump: The wound where his leg had been removed 20 years earlier had degenerated over time, so he had to have a bit of the stump re-amputated and a fresh stump with healthy tissue created.

drink. He was on the way to The Snout and Trotter, a small pub in the middle of prime pig land 80 km north of Adelaide. Twonames had been hit by a beer truck out the front of The Snout and Trotter when he was 18. An out-of-court settlement seemed to involve little more than medical expenses and free beer for the rest of his life.

We jerked and jumped up the road until Twonames had forced the unwilling Corona to get into 4th gear. It did seem odd that Twonames would own a manual and not an automatic. Three pedals, one leg. Didn't seem like great planning. We chatted, which was fun because Twonames heard about 50% of what I said and I understood about 50% of what he said. According to probability, this means that the conversation was actually four times as interesting as it appeared to be[22], and, as it was, it appeared to be quite interesting.

I did pick up that Twonames' favourite subject of discussion was his sister, of whom he was obviously proud. Unlike Twonames, she had made it right through school and now worked as a nurse at Townsville Base Hospital. "She got all the brains, I just got my mum's ears". Granted - they were absolute radar dishes (which made his hearing loss even more astounding), but they didn't seem all that out of place on the side of his head, which looked as though it could only have been plonked on top of his torso as a sort of after-thought: "Jeepers George, we need a head here – what've you got?" His face looked like it belonged on something far bigger than his body. A bonsai head. No neck to speak of and a tiny mouth that seemed to sit too low on his face. Despite the confronting nature of his appearance, he was as friendly a man as you could hope to meet, especially if you were hitch-hiking. Twonames spoke mainly in take-home messages, moral of the story's and tiny tit-bit's, the meaning of them was never obvious:

---

22 Probability: There may be a slight flaw in this reasoning.

"The moral of the story is don't swim with stingers unless you're a pack of salt & vinegar crisps"

or

"If you're goin' to sleep around, make sure you pack a few mozzie coils".

I was lucky enough to receive many tiny tit-bits during the time we had, none more impressive than the rationale behind keeping a bottle of beer in one's crotch. I had noticed early on that a six-pack of XXXX[23] that sat between the seats was missing one bottle. Not long in, he reached one hand up his faded blue shorts and pulled out the missing bottle. Needless to say I was interested in this. I asked him why he kept a beer up his shorts. It so happened that his sister, the nurse (who got all the brains), rang him excitedly in the middle of studying for her biology exam because she had just learnt that the whole reason men have scrotums in which to store their testicles is that it keeps the testicles cool and thereby ensures the health of the sperm. Twonames was noticeably impressed even as he recounted the fact:

"That's it! No other reason! Here's a tiny tit-bit for yer – it's not just for looks!"

Having done Human Systems 101 myself I was well aware of the need to keep the testicles below 40°C and that to keep them outside of our abdomen in a purpose-built sack seemed an ingenious way to do it. Twonames was on a roll and made me a generous offer:

---

23 XXXX: 'Four X' is a Queensland beer. Outside of Queensland, it is known as cow urine.

"The take home message is that you can use my scrotum to keep all sorts of things cool."

Mental note: do not share his egg sandwich.

I couldn't tell him that his sister had misunderstood the whole scrotum-testicles thing, I didn't have the heart. The other reason is that we arrived at The Snout and Trotter. Violently.

It was a pretty unimpressive pub, although it had a brand new car park. In fact, they had redesigned their carpark while Twonames was in hospital, which meant that when he drove in, at the same spot at which he would always drive in, we bounced up the gutter and crashed through a small hedge to stop in the bay between two big smelly waste bins. Twonames cursed something I couldn't quite understand, turned off the engine and sat shaking his head as though someone had just died. It was then that he freaked me out a second time.

Without any warning, a brutal look of raw and unadulterated fear took hold of his face. He swore and jumped back, clutching the cloth of the seat with rapidly-whitening knuckles. His eyes seemed to be locked on the clutch pedal. He was screaming blue murder and yelling at me:

Twonames: *"Me leg! Get me leg! Stick me leg on! Holy Mother of Jamie Wilson! Get me fuckin' leg! I gotta have me leg on!"*

Despite the clear sentiment of what he was saying, it took me a little while to get the message. He wanted me to put his prosthetic leg back where it should be. A bit perplexed and still unconvinced that Twonames hadn't seen the Ghost of Jamie Wilson's mother, I put his leg down on top of the clutch pedal, rested its top end at his stump and

53

adjusted it a bit so it looked to be on the right angle. However, that wasn't enough, Twonames was still writhing, now grabbing his prosthetic knee and looking at the foot.

> Twonames: "Take off me sock! Take off me bloody sock! Holy Mother of Jamie Wilson!! Me sock! Me sock!"

This Jamie Wilson fellow must have a really bad mother. Now Twonames was holding a screwdriver toward me and as I took the sock off I realised what the screwdriver was for and that neither Jamie Wilson, nor his mother, were relevant. There, on the outside of the top of his prosthetic foot was a little circle, about a centimetre in diameter, drawn in green marker. Next to the circle was the word "here" and an arrow pointing into the middle of the circle.

> Twonames: "Press me foot! Diggit into me foot! Move your arm you idiot – I gotta see it! I gotta see it!!"

No sooner had I dug the screwdriver into the well-worn spot on the top of his prosthetic foot than Twonames let out a moan of relief. The blood returned to his face and he loosened his grip on his prosthetic knee.

Obviously, I was intrigued by this. Half of me was thinking 'what a complete joker' and half of me was thinking 'how amazing is that?!?' It was like his rubber foot was actually hurting.' I asked him:

> LM: What on earth was going on there?'
> Twonames: "That has been happening ever since I lost the leg. Twenny years. I get this sudden, burning, white hot, shooting pain in me foot, travels up the front of me shin where it digs into me knee and feels like it will blow me whole leg into a million pieces. It is murder. Bloody murder. They used to have to strap me down when I was

younger. Knock me out. Everyone thought I was going crazy – 'specially me – I thought I was going completely nuts. Only discovered by accident that if I have me rubber leg on, I could turn the pain clear off by pressing something really hard into that spot on the top. That's the spot where I was pinned down when the truck hit me. Dunno why that matters, but apparently it does. I don't know why digging a screwdriver into it turns the pain off 'n' it doesn't work if I can't see it, but if I can see it, it's just like a switch. A magic bloody button. Beautiful".

With that, Twonames threw me back the leg and said

"Coming in for a lager? It's on them. I'd rather hop – will yer bring me leg?"

so what has Twonames and his magic button got to do with pain?

The one sentence take home message: It hurts where your brain *thinks* the problem is, not necessarily where the problem really is.

There are a couple of things that I think are groovy about his story.

1. Twonames had no leg, but he still got pain in his leg. What's more, he still got pain in his leg 20 years after his leg had been removed. What's more, the worst pain he had, that burning 'white-hot' pain, was felt in the same place that he had been pinned down all those years ago. Pain in an amputated or

55

missing body part is known as phantom limb pain and it is reasonably common. It can be associated with any missing body part. In fact, you don't even have to have ever had the body part for it to hurt. That the brain is able to make a missing limb hurt, and make the pain as intense, as bad and as real as it does when the leg is actually there, shows me that it is the brain that makes things hurt.

2.   Phantom limb pain also shows me that despite the fact that Twonames knew for a fact that he had no leg – there is not an ounce of doubt about it – his brain still made his leg hurt. In order to do this, the brain must have a map of the body that it uses to give us bodily feelings, including pain. We know that this is the case and there are ways to measure where in the brain different body maps are held. We know that every single bodily feeling we ever had is constructed by the brain and 'projected' onto a virtual body. Thus, it is the virtual body, or the maps of the real body, that determine where things hurt. This doesn't always coincide with what is actually happening in the body. That is obvious for Twonames, but there are other examples that are less drastic, like leg pain related to danger messages coming from the back. The brain mistakenly 'projects' the pain onto the virtual leg. Try telling someone with burning leg pain that their pain isn't real and they will more than likely biff you one. The leg pain is 100%, completely, undeniably, real, even though there is nothing at all wrong with the leg.

3.   The way that Twonames could eliminate his pain, very quickly, was by digging a screwdriver into a spot on his rubber leg that felt like the source of his pain, so long as he could see it happen. I have no idea why digging a screwdriver in made the pain stop, but there is a bunch of stuff that shows how the brain can use visual information to modify bodily feelings. It was crucial that the brain saw the leg and saw that something had been done. That shows me that the virtual body part can still be modified even though the real body part is missing. That, I reckon, is superb.

scratchy & the boring talker (the snake bite stories)

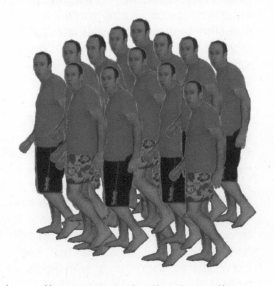

Or: Pain depends on the answer to the question
"How dangerous is this *really?*"

Or: Pain depends on experience

1. Scratchy

About two hours south of Sydney, in the superb southern tablelands, is Wollondilly River. Our mates PC and Kaz have a little block of land there. They call their block of land Rivendell. It is indeed God's Country – yellow box and river gums, tough granite outcrops and knee high bush grass. Not a sound aside from the natural inhabitants. Kookaburras, Whoopee birds[24], Koalas. Koalas do not sound nearly as cute as they look. They actually sound a bit like a neglected Skoda SuperSport 110 (see chapter called Nigel's skoda) – a throaty, almost raspy, growl. It is a noise, not a call. Furthermore it is a noise that is not nice. It is a little frightening if you don't know what it is and only slightly less frightening if you do, because you can't believe such a devilish groan can emerge from such a cute cuddly sleepy animal.

As the crow flies, Rivendell is not too far from civilisation. As the four wheel drive drives, it is. PC and Kaz spend most weekends there and love to have visitors. PC is one of those blokes who just loves to be nude. In fact he loves to be *nooode*. What's more, he loves his *nooode-ness* in that *jiggly-wiggly* kind of way. Apparently he takes off his gear as soon as their 4WD crosses the boundary into their land and doesn't put it back on until their 4WD crosses the boundary back out. The exception to the *jiggly-wiggly nooode* policy is when he has visitors who might be less comfortable than he is with jiggly-wiggly, or nooode, or both. Visitors, for example, like us.

We visited PC and Kaz one weekend in May. It was a glorious time of year – a chill coming into the air, but crisp sunny mornings and calm cool evenings. We had a lovely evening chatting about *stuff*. With PC and Kaz, a Cab Sav conversation was always around the corner and a surprisingly refreshing aspect was that it was always PC

---

24 Whoopee birds: I suspect this is not their official zoological name.

talking. About himself, primarily, but in an interesting and reflective way. We all enjoyed the genuine wonder he got when he contemplated himself.

Next morning I got up with the sun and donned my *sarong*. Very groovy indeed. PC and Kaz and TMBA[25] were still asleep, so I tiptoed outside and strolled down toward the river, which was more of a creek really. It was a splendid morning. I love dawn. Everything is still. The birds are active but the koalas are not. I love knowing that most people are asleep, as though all this magnificent beauty is there for just me to enjoy. I shuffled down the slope, just in my sarong and a t-shirt. I could feel the soft sand squeezing up between my toes and the crunchy dry grass and shrubs prickling my ankles. I remember, vaguely, a sharper prickling slightly beyond my ankle – sharp enough to make me flick my foot, let out a tiny 'ooh' and squint my eyes a fraction. That was it. Let me tell you, by way of a very bad picture and some lines, what I think happened in that moment, from a biological perspective. Make sure you start at the bottom box, numbered 1.

---

[25] TMBA: The most beautiful Anna, with whom I share my life & my children.

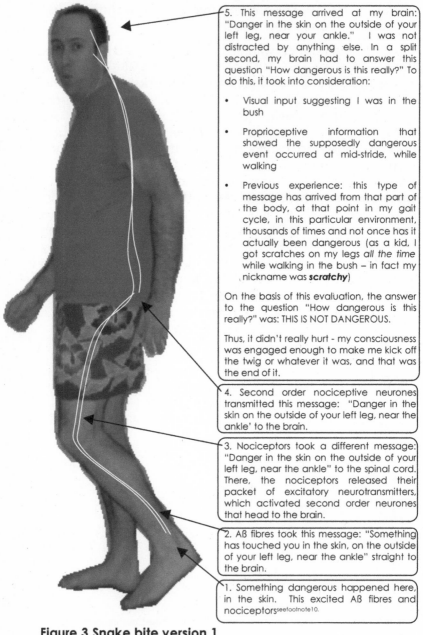

5. This message arrived at my brain: "Danger in the skin on the outside of your left leg, near your ankle." I was not distracted by anything else. In a split second, my brain had to answer this question "How dangerous is this really?" To do this, it took into consideration:

- Visual input suggesting I was in the bush

- Proprioceptive information that showed the supposedly dangerous event occurred at mid-stride, while walking

- Previous experience: this type of message has arrived from that part of the body, at that point in my gait cycle, in this particular environment, thousands of times and not once has it actually been dangerous (as a kid, I got scratches on my legs *all the time* while walking in the bush – in fact my nickname was ***scratchy***)

On the basis of this evaluation, the answer to the question "How dangerous is this really?" was: THIS IS NOT DANGEROUS.

Thus, it didn't really hurt - my consciousness was engaged enough to make me kick off the twig or whatever it was, and that was the end of it.

4. Second order nociceptive neurones transmitted this message: "Danger in the skin on the outside of your left leg, near the ankle' to the brain.

3. Nociceptors took a different message: "Danger in the skin on the outside of your left leg, near the ankle" to the spinal cord. There, the nociceptors released their packet of excitatory neurotransmitters, which activated second order neurones that head to the brain.

2. Aß fibres took this message: "Something has touched you in the skin, on the outside of your left leg, near the ankle" straight to the brain.

1. Something dangerous happened here, in the skin. This excited Aß fibres and nociceptors[see footnote 10].

Figure 3 Snake bite version 1

You have probably guessed that the dangerous thing that happened was a snake bite. No ordinary snake mind you – an Eastern Brown. Eastern Brown snakes are notoriously good. At killing. This is what Wikipedia (www.wikipedia.com) says about the Eastern Brown:

> The **Eastern Brown Snake** is the second most venomous land snake in the world after the Inland Taipan. Although an Eastern Brown will seek to avoid a confrontation, it has a very toxic venom, and.....have been known to cause fatalities in humans. The venom contains both neurotoxins and blood coagulants.

My mate Chris Jackson was incredulous that something with a brain the size of a pea could knock off a human. I wonder what he thought about box jellyfish[26]. I think he would take issue with Wikipedia's conservation classification of the Eastern Brown as an animal of 'least concern'[27].

The overwhelming response to surviving a bite from such an animal is something like 'my giddy aunt that was close!' But there is a sequel to the snake bite story. It occurred about 6 months later. I was walking again in a National Park inside Sydney. Lane Cove national park. One of the many things I love about Sydney is that it is such a *beautiful* city. It really is. Not just for its harbour, which is appropriately famous, nor for its beaches, which are also pretty well known, but also for the unsung national parks within its

---

26 Box jellyfish: The box jellyfish is also lethal and has no central nervous system. Jacko would *hate* that.

[27] Of least concern refers to the remote chance that the Eastern Brown will ever become extinct.

boundaries. There is Royal National Park at the southern end of Sydney. From the northern end of the Royal NP one can sit and watch the jumbos come into Kingsford Smith Airport and Sydney city's tallest buildings are clearly visible in the background. Two hundred and thirty years ago the original Australians would have stood in the exact same place and watched in wonder at the Endeavour and its fleet as they washed into Botany Bay. Overdressed pale-skinned men, as badly suited to this country as it is possible to be, would have been staring back in equal wonder at the unfamiliar landscape of 'Terra Australis'. One can walk for two days in Royal National Park, never be more than 20 km from the CBD and only meet the occasional fellow walker. I love Sydney.

This one fine November day however, I was walking in Lane Cove National Park. Lane Cove NP is less than 10 km from the CBD and about half way between the coast, a natural barrier to Sydney's eastward expansion, and Sydney's geographical centre. Once in the park, one can easily become convinced that the urban sprawl is miles away, even though it is literally surrounding them, less than a kilometre away in most directions.

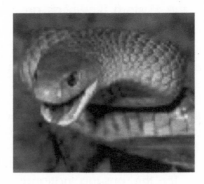

Figure 4 Just like the nasty customer that got me

It is important for this story to point out that I was walking with a small party, one of whom was a boring-talker. Everyone knows a boring-talker, although they may never have realised it. Boring-talkers are those people who, no matter what they are talking *about*, make it completely and utterly *boring*. Bores you almost to tears. Well I know one such Boring-talker, who I will refer to as Helen. That is not her real name. In my talks I use her real name but she might just read this, so I have called her Helen. I so-happened to be in a conversation with boring-talker as we were walking along the windy track through Lane Cove NP. She was talking about something, but as it is impossible to remember anything without attending to it, and as it is impossible to attend to a boring-talker, I don't remember what Helen was talking about. I do remember that she was talking, because I remember having to reply every few seconds with a "Right" or an "OK", with the occasional 'Really? Wow!"[28]

Anyway, as I was walking, I remember, this time quite clearly, feeling a really sharp prickling pain on the outside of my left leg, just above the ankle. If I was distracted I may not have felt it. Distraction remains our strongest analgesic. However, thanks to Helen, I was not distracted!

The pain was immediate and really intense. It was an electric, burning sensation that quite literally took my breath away. The pain shot up my leg like an electric bolt. It really *really* hurt. I couldn't help but yell out, partly I think in shock but then in pain. I doubled over, fell backward onto a conveniently situated rock and gripped my leg. I couldn't stop my face from contorting and my eyes switching between looking for the snake like a madman for sanity, and then clamping tight. I was in agony.

I hadn't just *imm*obilised myself. I had mobilised the rest of the walking party. They were all attending to me. Jacko was on his mobile phone (the other side of having a National Park in the middle of the city) to the ambulance

28 "Right. OK. Really!? WOW!": Let's be honest, we have all done this more than once.

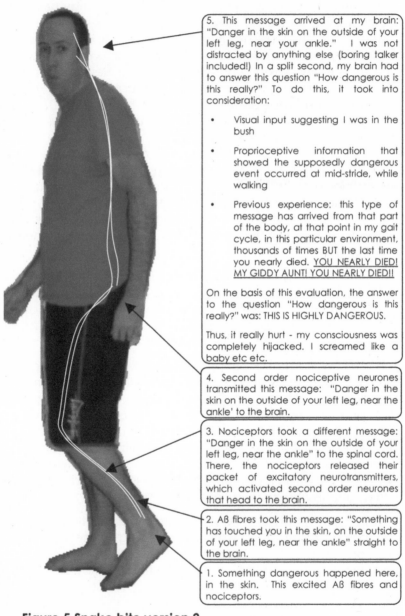

5. This message arrived at my brain: "Danger in the skin on the outside of your left leg, near your ankle." I was not distracted by anything else (boring talker included!) In a split second, my brain had to answer this question "How dangerous is this really?" To do this, it took into consideration:

- Visual input suggesting I was in the bush

- Proprioceptive information that showed the supposedly dangerous event occurred at mid-stride, while walking

- Previous experience: this type of message has arrived from that part of the body, at that point in my gait cycle, in this particular environment, thousands of times BUT the last time you nearly died. YOU NEARLY DIED! MY GIDDY AUNT! YOU NEARLY DIED!!

On the basis of this evaluation, the answer to the question "How dangerous is this really?" was: THIS IS HIGHLY DANGEROUS.

Thus, it really hurt - my consciousness was completely hijacked. I screamed like a baby etc etc.

4. Second order nociceptive neurones transmitted this message: "Danger in the skin on the outside of your left leg, near the ankle' to the brain.

3. Nociceptors took a different message: "Danger in the skin on the outside of your left leg, near the ankle" to the spinal cord. There, the nociceptors released their packet of excitatory neurotransmitters, which activated second order neurones that head to the brain.

2. Aß fibres took this message: "Something has touched you in the skin, on the outside of your left leg, near the ankle" straight to the brain.

1. Something dangerous happened here, in the skin. This excited Aß fibres and nociceptors.

Figure 5 Snake bite version 2

service: "Hurry! We have a bloke here who has been bitten by a snake, he has a minute to live!"[29]   Helen, I think, may still have been talking. Not sure. It wasn't for a couple of minutes that anyone had a close inspection of the area, at which time we realised that I had indeed been scratched by a twig. There was a single, tiny scratch mark on my leg. I have drawn here another picture of what I think happened this time, biologically.

The thing is, the first time, it didn't really hurt. The second time, it did. It *really* hurt. More than that, the first time I had groin pain for about a week. The second time I had recurrent aches in my groin for about a week. This was after I *knew* it was a scratch from a twig. It was as though my brain, at a deeper implicit level, wasn't convinced that I was completely safe from harm.

so, what do the snake bite stories tell us about pain?

The one sentence take home message: Pain depends on the brain's evaluation of how much danger you are *really* in.

I think pain is a pretty good indicator of the brain's perception of tissue danger. That is, I subscribe to the notion, which is not my notion, but one I think is the best, that pain can be considered the conscious correlate of the brain's implicit perception of how much danger the body part concerned is in. For different versions of this same notion, refer to the

---

29 "A minute to live!" I made up the mobile phone & ambulance call bit.

reference list at the back of this book. Another way of stating this, and the way I state it to patients, is that pain is determined by the brain's answer to this question:

"How dangerous is this?"

If the brain has received danger messages from the nerves in the body that are designed to detect danger, then the question becomes:

"How dangerous is this <u>really</u>?

So, going back to the first snake bite story, the brain received the danger messages loud and clear, but concluded that it was not *really* that dangerous. In the second scenario, the brain received danger messages from a similar location and concluded that the situation was potentially life threatening. What better way than undeniable agony to make me, the organism, limit the danger by:

(i)   stopping

(ii)   making everyone else stop

(iii)   taking the weight off the leg

(iv)   looking around for the snake, possibly to avoid a second bite, or to avoid another person getting bitten

It seems to me, to be a very effective system.

"How dangerous is this really?"

There are a few things about these stories that I point out to patients:

1. That the brain did all this evaluation outside of my consciousness and outside of my control.

2. That it happened in a split second.

3. That it happened to *me* when *I* spend 40 hours a week[30] *studying* this system. This is *what I do*. It is my job. And, despite that, my brain was still 'tricked'.

4. That I had pains in my groin for a week or so afterwards, even though I *knew* that it was a scratch and nothing to worry about. That I had those pains tells me that my brain was not convinced that there was indeed nothing to worry about. I find this point really useful with patients who are adamant in saying that they are quite happy to believe there is nothing wrong in their body. I use this example to demonstrate that there is a whole lot going on in your brain that you don't know about, and only a tiny amount that you do.

5. That the single experience in which I nearly died is enough to cause exquisite pain next time a similar situation occurs. This incredible adaptability is, I think, very cool. I tell patients that I think it is very cool too!

---

30 Working week: Truth be known it is probably only about 34 hours a week, but one must keep up appearances.

mr hammerhead shark

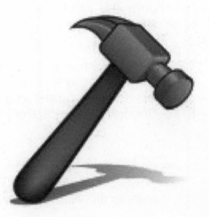

Or: Nociception is not sufficient for pain.

Royal North Shore Hospital was, for a long time, Sydney's biggest hospital. The emergency department had a huge waiting area, right next to where the ambulances would bring in the patients on those magic folding beds. I had noted the hospital's design on a previous visit as a patient, when I popped my shoulder out playing Australian Rules Football on a ground just out the front. I thought it intriguing that the waiting area would have full view of the ambulance chute. Wouldn't they want to keep it a bit private so that patients in the waiting area didn't have to watch those, with injuries too severe to come in themselves, writhe and moan as they went through to theatre? I presumed so, but as I sat there waiting for someone to return my arm from where it was (protruding out of what looked like a tumour about midway between my nipple and the point of my shoulder) to where it should have been, I noticed that none of the people who came in with the ambulance seemed to be writhing, or moaning. I thought this rather intriguing, so I took it upon myself to investigate this phenomenon more carefully once I was reshouldered.

A few weeks later (not *all* that time was spent waiting for my turn in the emergency room!), I packed a couple of salad sandwiches, a space food stick (caramel), a couple of apples and a popper[31] (orange and mango), and set off to Royal North Shore Hospital with this question in mind:

> *"What is the writhe and moan ratio between patients coming in the ambulance with severe injuries and those walking into Emergency with mild injuries?"*[32]

I compiled a little table that I thought would encapsulate the main pieces of data. The tricky thing was to ask the patient some questions without getting in trouble with the

---

31 Popper: a fruit juice in a small carton with a straw attached to the outside.

32 Original?: I have written this as though I was the first person to ever wonder about the relationship between injury severity and pain, which I wasn't. In fact, this relationship has been the subject of much writing, but I will still *pretend* I thought of it. In actual fact, it was just that I didn't really believe what I had read because it sounded rather stupid.

staff. I was particularly concerned about the chief triage nurse. He was a really big fellow with a face like a pitbull. I could not understand why they would put such an incredibly intimidating-looking person on triage – perhaps to sort those in genuine need from those just coming in for a chat. My fears about him were allayed somewhat when I heard him offer one patient a cup of tea, which he did in a high, very feminine-sounding singing voice – a bit like Tinkerbell meets Sound of Music. Nonetheless, I was keen to be as discrete as possible in asking patients the necessary questions to complete my table. I kept my clipboard with me and stuck my University Library card in a plastic wallet and clipped it to my shirt. I asked them what they had done and how much did it hurt. Here is my table. I have put some of what I wrote that day in there.

Injury	LM gory index	Writhe score	Moan score	Pain
Ingrown toenail	3	3	6	8
Dislocated & # knee (A)	7 (wrong)	2	0	2
Dislocated finger	4	4	2	4
Grazed leg	0	3	5	6
Hammer through neck	9 (v. wrong!)	0	0	0

The most remarkable patient was the last one. He came in through the emergency department, having been driven there by the thrower of the hammer. That same hammer was now inserted through the side of his neck. It looked filthy – the tips of the curly bit were just poking out of the front of his neck, having entered from the rear. As he walked across the waiting area, he held the handle of the hammer out at right angles. There were groans and moans from the rest of us as we watched him – he, on the other hand, was as happy as Larry. Here is a reasonably faithful transcript of our conversation:

LM: Crikey mate! What happened?

71

Man with hammer in neck: Classic isn't it?! Giorgio pretended to throw this hammer at me, which was a bit of fun, but he accidentally let go of the thing, which was a bit daft. Great shot but, wasn't it? Straight through me neck – I gotta hold it out to the side so it doesn't pull me off balance!

LM: Doesn't it hurt?

Man with hammer in neck: Na – that's the thing – it hurt when it went in but not that much – naagh, now it doesn't seem to hurt at all – must have missed all me main bits.

LM: Not at all? I mean it looks wrong.

Man with hammer in neck: Not at all – hey. I got this great gag – Giorgio reckons it's a classic.

At this, the man with a hammer in his neck bent over forward so that his torso was horizontal. He put his right hand on his hip and pointed his elbow up in the air. He moved is left hand around so as to stabilise the hammer and then shuffled across the waiting room in a zig-zaggy kind of way.

Man with hammer in neck: What am I? What am I?

LM: I have no idea. A complete nutter?

Man with hammer in neck: No, no – think about it! What am I?

LM: (Giggling a little embarrassingly) I don't know.

Man with hammer in neck: Der der….Der der…..Der der

(At this point I need to tell you that the der der der der der der is my way of telling you that he did that noise from JAWS, when everyone was

72

swimming in the water and you just knew that the mega-shark was getting close etc etc.)

Anyway, continuing on....

Der di Der di..........I'm a hammer-head shark yer goose!

At that, Giorgio cracked up completely and had to sit down. Most people in the waiting room were laughing, except one guy who had more or less passed out at the sight of this fellow with a hammer hanging out of his neck playing charades in the waiting room.

But here is the coolest bit – Mr Hammerhead shark spun around and hit his knee on the end of a table, at which he promptly swore and hobbled onto a seat, holding his knee, grimacing and saying:

"Shit! My knee! Shit shit shit! Ow! Shit! SHIT!"

The pitbull triage nurse was alerted by the waiting room commotion and then excited by the expletives. He looked up, saw a man with a hammer sticking out of his neck, sang "golly goonda my aunt jane" just like a Fairy Godmother might, called for the wardman and ran over to attend to Mr Hammerhead. There they were, the triage nurse, foaming at the mouth, looking like the front end of a woolly mammoth but sounding like Tinkerbell,, and a man with a hammer stuck in his neck. Tinkerbell was waving his hands about singing "Don't move your head! Don't move your head!" while Mr Hammerhead was shouting at the top of his voice "It's my friggin' knee you moron! My friggin' knee!"

so, what has mr hammerhead got to do with pain?

The one sentence take home message: Danger to your tissues doesn't always mean it will hurt.

There are two reasons that this story makes it into many of my sessions with patients. The first is that it is funny. At least I reckon it's funny and most patients tend to at least get a giggle out of it. I find that getting a giggle makes the patient and me feel a bit more comfortable with each other. The second reason is that it is a perfect example of <u>the fact</u> that nociception is not sufficient for pain. It was not that Mr Hammerhead had no *ability* to feel pain, nor that he was temporarily rendered euphoric by circulating chemicals in his bloodstream (stress-induced analgesia). Those two things are ruled out by his outrageous response when he knocked his knee on the table.

It is not that the hammer would have missed nociceptors[33] when it went through his neck. On the contrary, there are thousands of nociceptors that would have been activated by the hammer. So much so that they would have, as we say in the scientific literature, gone bezerk.

So, despite nociceptors going bezerk, Mr Hammerhead had no pain.

Everyone has stories like this – I don't have any that are as funny, but there is no doubt that this sort of thing happens in one form or another to most of us. *Explain Pain* has many amazing pain stories that show us that **nociception is not sufficient for pain.** That is the main message of Mr

---

33 A nociceptor: Nociceptor is the term given to nerve cells in your body that respond to dangerous things. To learn about how they work and the role they have in pain, read *Explain Pain*, which is in the reference list at the back of this book.

Hammerhead's story I think – that nocieption is not enough. In order to experience pain, the brain has to

(i)   conclude that tissue is in danger, and

(ii)   conclude that you, the organism, should *do* something about it.

ant fettuccine

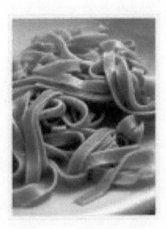

Or: Nociception is neither sufficient nor necessary
for pain

The Beautiful Anna, with whom I share my life, once got an ant in her ear. How this happened is somewhat of a mystery. One minute she was walking along as she had always been – 'ant-free' – and the next minute there was

77

something scratching around in her ear. Neither of us knew it to be an ant, that became clear somewhat later on. I have never had an ant in my ear, but by all appearances it is a rather distressing experience. At first it was annoying, primarily because it was so loud, which I guess it would be because it is walking over your eardrum.

We tried several means to get it out. I got Anna to shake her head violently from side to side as you might if you had a grasshopper in your hair. I tried to tempt it out by balancing a crisp on Anna's earlobe and ruffling the packet. This I called the picnic approach. I even tried the vacuum cleaner. Anna lay on the couch with her ant-ear facing up. I placed my index finger over the edge of her ear hole so as to avoid the Hoover nozzle creating a seal and sucking her brains out[34]. The plan was that I would hold the nozzle vertically over her head and slowly move it closer and closer until she felt the little bugger stop his hanging on for dear life and slip up the ear canal like a beetle on the windscreen. We figured you would hear it scraping and possibly making a few little yelping-type noises.

Funnily enough, none of our attempts were successful, although several times we thought it must have worked because the little bugger would be silent for a while. Anna would start to relax, wobble her head around a little and as soon as she said "I think it might be out" an almost deafening scrape or whack would tell her otherwise.

It was not long before Anna's ear began to hurt – a diffuse dull ache that slowly spread over a fair portion of the right side of her head. We began to wonder if this creature might have bitten her, or stung her and that perhaps the poison was starting to have an effect. She began to hold her head tilted a bit to the right and turned back a little. Her right shoulder started to lift up and come forward a

---

34 Suck your brains out: OK OK OK, I know that you can't *really* suck your brains out via your ear and that you would be more likely to inflict damage on the ear apparatus, but it sounds so much better to say 'suck your brains out'. Suck your brains out. See?

little. Her posture was just like that posture you adopt when someone tries to poke you just behind your collar bone. Her right eye started to squint a little and her mouth tightened up just a touch on that side.

As time progressed, the dull ache became stronger. It would become worse when she put her head down or moved it too quickly. It was time to see a doctor. We jumped in the car and drove to the local hospital. On entering the emergency department, we were quickly attended to by a charming fellow in a white coat, confident yet caring voice. There was no waiting for us this time. Despite there being several people in the waiting room, it seemed that obvious head pain or trauma gets prioritised. This is what our doctor said:

> *Doctor: OK. What's wrong with your head – there is obviously something going on. Is it your ear?* (very encouraging)
>
> *TBA: Yes, there is something, I think, in my right ear – I thought it might be a bug or something, but now the whole right side of my head hurts.*
>
> *Doctor: OK. Probably an ant. Lie down here with that ear facing up.*

Anna promptly followed his instructions and waited. He snuck into a nearby examination room. That he snuck in there did seem a bit odd but we quickly disregarded his sneakingness. He came back with a little bottle of olive oil.

> *Doctor: I am just going to pour a little olive oil into your ear.   Remain   still   for   about   30 seconds.................OK. now sit up and tilt your head right over to the right.*

With this, he held a bowl under Anna's right ear and a small amount of olive oil dribbled into it and there, in the olive oil was a dead ant. The relief on Anna's face was obvious. She wiggled her head, moved her jaw up and down a little and we both turned to the doctor, who was holding the bowl and looking proudly into it as though he had just given birth to the ant.

> *Doctor: There's the little blighter — just like the one we had in here the other day. They must love the ear canal perhaps. I might cook up some pasta next time — ant fettuccine!*
>
> *Anna: Thank you so much! And thanks for seeing me so soon. Do I need to fill out any forms or give in my insurance details or anything?*
>
> *Doctor: I think so. Perhaps you should see a doctor anyway?*

This was somewhat surprising to us both.

> *Anna & LM: But aren't you the doctor!?*
>
> *No longer doctor: Oh no, no. I am here to see one too.*

With this, the fellow walked across the waiting room with a big limp, as big as you might have if you had a wooden leg two sizes too big. Indeed, on the bottom of his right foot was a big lump of wood. His shoe was stained bright crimson with blood and poking out the top was a big fat nail. This man, who we thought to be the doctor, who was charming and confident and calm throughout our ant in the ear ordeal, had a piece of wood nailed to his foot.

LM (thinking quickly): You've got a lump of wood nailed to your foot!

No longer doctor: I know! Amazing isn't it – nail gun – straight through, nailed my foot to the floor! Had to cut the floor up to get in here. I walked over from the other side of the highway (about a kilometre) *– save the taxi fare – those bastards charge a couple of bucks just to get up in the morning!*

so, what has ant fettuccine got to do with pain?

The one sentence take home message: Pain doesn't always mean there is tissue in danger.

This story follows the last one because it does more than demonstrate that nociception is not sufficient for pain (as evidenced by the man we thought was a doctor, who had nailed his foot to the floor and was experiencing no pain). Actually, this scenario is an example that nociception is not necessary for pain. TMBA probably had no nociceptive input when the ant was in her ear. However, her head was starting to hurt and her muscles had started to protect that side of her head. Thus, nociception is neither sufficient, nor necessary, for pain.

There are also some really interesting experiments that show that nociception is not sufficient for pain. Here is the most cheeky experiment: Researchers convinced subjects to put their heads in what they called a 'head stimulator'. When the researchers turned up the intensity knob, the subjects reported that their head started to hurt. What's more, pain ratings related to the intensity settings. That might not seem

81

surprising, except that the stimulator wasn't real – it wasn't even connected to the control knobs! [Ref List No. 5]

dusty's bum crack.

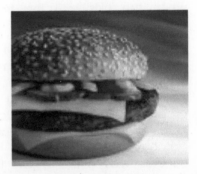

Or: the brain samples information according to
perceived vulnerability and threat.

When I was in high school, around about that time I first
encountered Mrs Smart and the visual perception system, I
got a job at the local McDonalds. It was a great job, not
least for the seemingly endless variety of injury-free

practical jokes one could play on colleagues and on customers. I was particularly fond of putting 3 or 4 fish fillet's in a Fillet-o-fish© burger and watch the absolute ecstasy on the face of whoever bought it when they opened the lid. I could fit 13 nuggets in a six-pack, although you had to hold the lid down and pass it over (to my dad, usually) in that way. Otherwise, the lid would pop open and, as they say, there would be some explaining to do.

McDonalds stores are divided into two bits – the front and the back. When referring to 'the back' or 'the front', you had to preface it with 'out'. For example, 'out the back' was where the boys worked and 'out the front' was where the girls worked, except the ugly or angry girls, who worked on drive-through, or possibly on salad. It was a job of the boys 'out the back' to keep the products available so that when the girls 'out the front' received an order, the customer never had to wait.

The most important job 'out the back' was 'Production'. In that job, you had to keep an eye on the customers and on the supply, so that you never ran out of product. However, you had to avoid being overstocked too, because products were not allowed to spend more than 15 minutes in the production chute. One put a timer in behind each batch so that they would be thrown out when the 15 minutes was over.[35] On Production, you would bark requests at the other pimply-faced youths out the back – each one of them in charge of a station – big macs©, salad, fries, grill, gofer[36]. The most demanding station was quarter pounders©. Only those blokes who had demonstrated their ability, in the midst of a busload of

---

35 Production at McDonalds: Of course in reality, the true champions at the job of Production were only champions because they could keep changing the timers without anyone noticing, so that they never had to throw anything out. I made a point of not doing this, partly because I was afraid of giving someone a bacteria burger and partly because I was afraid of getting caught.

36 Gofer: The 'gofer' was the general tasks person, the dog's body. Called gofer because they go for this and go for that.

school kids or a university ski trip, to get the job done, were ever put on quarter pounders. Those who demonstrated they could cope with quarter pounders in the rush, were then eligble for production. This promotional criterion was not official, but it was how it worked.

One day I arrived at work and saw my roster – production. I was reasonably chuffed with that, not because it is the captain's gig, but because it was one of about three spots in which your clothes didn't become toxic over the course of a shift. 'Fat pants' was particularly nasty on 'Grill'. You could wear two aprons over your shirt and pants, and you would still get greasy fat-blisters on your legs by the end of a shift. I was as pleased about getting Production as I was disappointed that Dusty got Quarter pounders. Dusty had worked in our store longer than I had but had the misfortune of being (i) the son of the manager and (ii) crap at Quarter pounders. Dusty knew he was no good at Quarter pounders, but because he was the manager's son, he was too afraid to refuse the shift when the manager rostered him on. He was even too afraid to swap stations when a busload arrived. Instead, he would duck off to the toilet. Bad strategy.

Being on Production when Dusty was on quarter pounders was bad news. I kept a particularly close eye on quarter pounders – I scanned the environment for customers that *looked* like they might be quarter pounder eaters (not that I really knew what they looked like, but I was hoping that I would recognise them when they appeared). I kept an eye on how many meat patties Dusty was putting down on the grill. Everytime I barked him an order –

"can I have 6 turn-lay quarter pounders please Dusty"

Dusty would reply with:

"6 turn-lay quarter pounders, thank you production".

I took special notice of whether or not he implemented this instruction.

In this manner, the evening passed fairly uneventfully, although I did end up over-requesting quarter pounders a couple of times and having to dump them when they passed the timers. I think my action was justified, particularly when one family, fat mum fat dad and two fat kids, waddled in, t-shirts that said:

> *"My grampa went to Texas and all he got me was this lousy T-shirt (and a semi-automatic shotgun)".*

I thought these guys were sure-fire Quarterpounder eaters. That I over-compensated for Dusty's anticipated vulnerability is evidence that, before he had even stuffed up, I was changing my behaviour, and changing the way the whole body of staff were working. I did all of this to protect the store.

But then the inevitable happened – three buses of hungry uni students on the way home after a weekend of skiing. Not wanting to overwhelm Dusty, I upped the request slowly:

> *LM: "9 turn-lay Quarter pounders please Dusty"*
>
> *Dusty: "9 turn-lay Quarter pounders thank you production"*

Suffice to say, Dusty fell apart. Quarter pounders came out so raw that one kid complained that there was water in his ketchup when blood was oozing down the bun. Some burgers had no slices of cheese, others had extra slices. The production chute was empty and Dusty was completely flustered until he left 24 patties burning on the grill and went to the toilet (such was his habit in times of stress). Such a malfunction imposes a serious threat to the whole place – customers get angry and impatient, workers get testy, the whole place gets messy, pickles on the floor, rubbish bins overflowing, Drive-thru traffic banks up, etc etc. I took solace in the fact that the store would eventually close for the night and, ultimately, we all knew that Dusty was at the bottom of it all.

It was months before I was again faced with the misfortune of doing Production when Dusty was on Quarter pounders. This time, however, I had strategies in place to help minimise the impact. This is what I did:

(i)   I had the drive-through staff be on alert for buses, so as to get some early warning.

(ii)   I had the guy on Nuggets keep a look out for Dusty's bum crack – loss of altitude on the pantline was the first sign that Dusty was starting to lose it.

(iii)   I had the girl on Salad keep a look out for Dusty's stress rash that started beneath his left ear and slowly crept around his neck like an Amish beard.

(iv)   I planted a note on the crew room toilet door that said "Bathroom undergoing emergency repairs – see Lorimer for alternative key".

All of these things were ways in which I had increased the likelihood of detecting something starting to go amiss on Dusty's station. The strategy worked pretty well in so far as we didn't run out of food and the place *seemed* to keep operating fairly normally. However, it meant that there were some false alarms. It meant I had fewer resources to allocate to other jobs. It meant that we had to throw away more food than usual. Occasionally, those people who were working extra hard to compensate for Dusty, to protect the entire process from Dusty's vulnerability, started getting grumpy. They also started slipping up themselves and the whole mood of the place headed south. As they say, a bad mood is a bad move.

Dusty didn't last long enough at McDonalds to get three gold stickers on his name badge. He had two golds (salad and fish fillets – very uncool) and a silver (dining room – even more uncool). Dusty convinced his dad, the store owner and manager, that he should have the jurisdiction to fire people. His dad reluctantly agreed and Dusty fired himself. "Gee that felt good" he said as he gave himself the marching orders and responded back to himself with the two fingered salute.

so, what has dusty's bum crack got to do with pain?

The one sentence take home message: If the brain perceives a part of your body is vulnerable, then it will protect it in every way it can, which may become a problem.

I use this story to talk about two aspects of what the brain does when it perceives a part of the body is vulnerable.

First, the brain implements strategies that protect that body part. Those strategies include changing the way the brain scans for threatening cues, using other body parts and systems to protect the area, moving slightly differently, behaving differently, avoiding some movements, activities and situations that might worsen the situation, reacting quickly at the first sign of danger, laying down more receptors for certain chemicals or stimuli.

Second, this is ultimately unsustainable. It leads to false alarms, over-reactions and break down of other body parts and systems. It prevents the vulnerable bit from becoming strong or more effective because it is always preventing that part being exposed to the threat. This is important because it is threat that promotes adaptation.

I also spend some time on the whole mood thing – to be protecting a vulnerable body part is stressful and chronic stress is a kill joy. The effects are substantial and widespread. *Why don't zebras get ulcers?* [Ref List No. 6] is a great account of the effects of long term stress.

ornithology & amazing grace

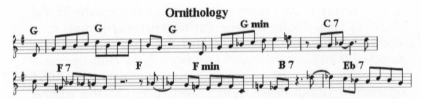

Or: neural networks that produce pain become
more sensitive when pain persists.

When I left physiotherapy school, I wanted to be a
musician. Not an obvious link and one that my dad
accepted bravely over a Super Supreme at Belfield Pizza
Hut. I remember it like it happened yesterday – Dad's oily

lips pursed together, a strand of mozzarella (or mozzarella-like imitation dairy product) clinging to his well-trimmed beard, his jaw muscles pulsating rhythmically. The fact is, I didn't want to be a physiotherapist. I had seen Cam Williams get coughed on through a tracheotomy and remember remnants of phlegm that were still wedged in the hinges of his glasses a week later. I had worn the sky-blue long socks that were required clinical uniform when I went through Uni[37]. I was not interested in doing that for a career. No no! I wanted to be a muso.

A critical issue that I had until then overlooked was that I had never played a musical instrument before. I had never had any type of music lesson and I had sold my unused recorder for some football cards as a kid. None-the-less, I got out the phone book and looked up

Music - Tuition — Brass - Saxophone

To my dismay there were no teachers of saxophone in the whole of New South Wales. On making this remark to a friend of mine, she explained that the saxophone was a woodwind instrument, which I thought quite daft because it is clearly not made of wood. She mumbled something incoherent about reeds and I went back to the phone book:

Music - Tuition — Woodwind - Saxophone

I have a policy of never selecting a business that has a boxed or bolded entry in the Yellow Pages. This policy is

---

37 Clinical uniform: I thought our socks were bad, but we were Milan compared to the girls. They had to wear the most abominable creations I have ever seen. They were called culottes:

culotte (kōō-lŏt') n. A woman's full trousers cut to resemble a skirt. Often used in the plural.

More accurately – 'a woman's full trousers cut to resemble a Yak.'

why I ended up knocking on the door of a dark, mouldy terrace in the rougher part of Petersham. Papa Smurf opened the door. Keith Silver. Keith Silver, Maestro. He *looked* a bit like Papa Smurf, but he had played saxophone with some of the best and I knew of him by reading the album covers of work by some of the best. Keith Silver thought that James Morrison was a rare talent who was predisposed to being a poser.

I figured that Keith Silver could recognise talent when he saw it. He didn't recognise me, which was disconcerting and probably should have been a 'Yellow Flag'. He stood at the door in his red and green tartan dressing gown, chewing on such a volume of Nicorette that his mouth looked like a harpsichord. Unfortunately, I had to remind him of our phone call and his promise to let me try before I buy. Memory jogged, he brought me into his studio and there sat an alto, a soprano, a base and, pride of place under spotlight, his Selmer Mk VI Tenor[38]. He gave me three reeds to suck on while he explained a couple of things about one's instrument being like a lover and that life was ultimately about music and sport and sport was for moron's, which made life about music. Sufficiently sogged, the reeds were inserted into each of the horns. He showed me how to hold it, and then how to blow it. I squeeked the soprano. I choked the bass. When I blew into the alto, there was no resistance, the wind just flew in and was replaced with this wonderful sound. I got the best part of a scale out of it and then ran out of air. "That", said Maestro, "is your horn". I was hooked. He didn't offer the Selmer, which is no surprise I guess.

A couple of months later Maestro started giving me technical exercises, which are specific tunes or passages of notes that one plays over and over and over again. The

---

38 Selmer Mk VI: If you haven't heard of a Selmer Mk VI, it is the ants pants, the bees knees, of saxophones – presents the serious muso with a real dilemma. I tried it on Keith:

> LM: *"Both the Mk VI and your daughter are stuck inside a burning house. You can only make one trip in..."*

idea is to get the fingers moving. I remember one exercise in particular because it led to my sacking from the only professional band I ever played in. It was a Charlie Parker tune called Ornithology[39]. Now, Charlie Parker, aka The Bird, to Jazz is like Rene Descartes to Pain sciences – both confronted the thought of the day head on and both totally revolutionised their world. I wanted to play Ornithology as fast, and as swinging, as The Bird. So, I played it to death – I played it during the day in the cupboard. I played it at night on Clovelly headland with seagulls, winos and young lovers for company. I played it until my lip bled and my octave thumb blistered. Ornithology rattled around in my brain like a bee in a bottle. It became *part* of me. The point is, I played the tune, the whole tune and, pretty much, nothing but the tune, for weeks. Months.

About a year later I had a regular gig as part of a five-piece jazz band. We played standards primarily and a few original tracks when the proprietor was too drunk to notice. One night someone in the club asked the band leader if she could sing with us. She was a beautiful black woman with a generous mouth and substantial curves – would have been hard to knock off her feet. She said 'corrl me Black Mama. Mazen Grace. Jerss farlo me borrs". She had a voice like chocolate and pretty soon we felt like a bonafide Gospel band - James Brown himself could have been in the house. Black Mama did some sublime scatting and the wonderful Amazing Grace theme bubbled around the band – double bass solo, piano solo, drum solo. Then me. I was, as they say, wailing. I had my sunglasses on. It was dark. I was dancing around a simple but stylish theme, fluttering and flirting irreverently with Amazing Grace. My mind wandered with the exploration – I could feel the wind

---

39 Ornithology: From when I got Ornithology to about 3 months before I wrote this, I thought Charlie Parker called his tune Hornithology, as a pun on the playing the horn. I was corrected by someone in a seminar I was running and I was so completely convinced that she was wrong that I made a joke of it. But she *was* right and *I* was wrong. If you read this, oh sufferer of the presenter's unjustified wrath, I am really sorry.

in my hair as together, the tune and I scampered across waves and over rock pools. Then it happened. Something unpredictable and uncontrollable occurred and I snapped without warning from Amazing Grace, straight into Ornithology. I was possessed by it. My fingers were flying! There I was, playing a perfectly tight Ornithology, right smack bang in the middle of Amazing Grace. It kept going – Ornithology had hijacked my body and my mind. Black Mama was staring at me with a look of 'what the -' The band leader was mouthing "what the – ?!" I was mouthing over the top of the sax "I don't f*!#$-ing know". I had no control over it – it was just *out there*. Everyone stopped playing except me. I stood there on stage, on my own, and finished Ornithology to the very end, even the tricky syncopated parts toward the end. The band-leader left a note in my sax-case:

You are a tosser and you are now out of work.

so, what have ornithology & amazing grace got to do with pain?

The one sentence take home message: When pain persists, it doesn't take much to make it hurt more.

The reason I tell people the Ornithology story is that I think it is a great metaphor for what happens when you are in pain for a long time. The metaphor draws on the idea of the brain being like an orchestra that can play many tunes (read *Explain Pain* to learn more about the idea of the brain being like an orchestra. I think the metaphor of the brain as an orchestra is really good and really useful).

The best theory we have at the moment of how pain emerges from the huge bundle of neurones that is your brain, is that something causes a particular network of neurones to activate. In *Explain Pain*, we call the network a neurotag. When the pain neurotag is activated, pain emerges. Playing Ornithology over and over and over again is like activating the pain neurotag over and over and over again. Cortical neurones, like spinal neurones, change when they are activated a lot. They become better at firing. In fact, they become so good at firing – so sensitive - that it becomes very difficult at times to identify what set them off. This means that pain can come on without warning, without control and without an obvious stimulus. Just like Ornithology did, in the middle of Amazing Grace.

Here is another example:

Men who have played a bit of cricket will relate to what happens when you see a batsman cop one in the grobbitz[40]. When I see this happen, I almost double over and I usually let out a groan as though in some way it is I who has been hit. A mate of mine played at the highest level and got belted several times, once when his protector had slipped out of position. He assured me that when he sees someone else get hit, it actually does hurt him – right inside the pelvic bones, which is where it hurts if you get hit. That visual information alone is enough to set off the pain neurotag is probably because his pain neurotag is sensitised to bits, or *hits* perhaps.

---

40 Grobbitz: That particular part of the male anatomy in which, or on which, one doesn't want to get hit. I remember Shane Warne getting middle-pegged by Freddy Flintoff in the now famous 2006 Ashes series (for which the entire English team (named so because at least 3 members were bonafide Englishmen) got Queen's honours (Paul Collingwood most famously, for his total of 7 runs) – shows that all one has to do for such things is to win a series every twenty years. Anyway, that is beside the point). When Warne had again taken up his stance at the batting crease, the commentator resumed in proper Kensington Plum "Flintoff to Warne, one ball left". Classic.

the hino story

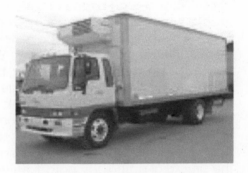

Or: Finding the angle in.

I drive trucks. I guess it is more accurate to say I drove trucks because I haven't been behind the wheel of a real truck for several years. I have *pretended* to be driving a truck with my boy Henry in my lap. We sometimes take the Volvo around the car park. We both really get into it – lean right over with one arm out the window and the other swivelling around the wheel. We both love putting on the air brake coming down Walton Well Road and of course releasing it when we stop – phffssssssssssssss-shooss!

I drove trucks for several years. I did supermarket deliveries and removalist work, picked up southern tablelands' potatoes for the Sydney fruit and veg markets, delivered pianos to simply-too-big houses in the Eastern Suburbs, transported cattle from one side of a property to the other. I did enough driving to get an idea of the idiosyncrasies of different types of trucks and the day-to-day life of someone who drives trucks. So what?

This experience behind the wheel came in handy one day when I was trying to get across the notion of *central sensitisation* to a group of patients, one of whom I was simply not *getting*. Before I go on with that story, let me talk about what I mean by the phrase to 'get someone'. This is exactly what TMBA would ask me, when I would return from a day at work 'Explaining pain' to patients with chronic pain problems:'did you get them?' By that she meant did I connect with them, did they buy the message, did I do whatever had to be done to 'get inside their heads'? Getting inside their head is, I think, critical if they are to consider information that is not consistent with what they have heard before, or with their own notion of what is happening inside their body. This is a difficult issue because the structural-pathology paradigm is alive and well in most western health care systems.

That is why I think it is critical to have an angle in, a way of communicating in the patient's language, a way of using a metaphor, a story, a *language* that the patient (i) finds interesting enough to listen to, (ii) is able to get involved with because it is accessible to them and their experiences, attitudes and beliefs, and (iii) is sufficiently so that they end up running with it and applying it to their own situation.

The truck driving story is one such situation – I was not winning with this fellow. He held a glazed look on his face

98

as though I really wasn't there. It is a remarkable capacity to engage sufficiently to know when one is being spoken to directly and to respond in a coherent and sensible way, but to be taking absolutely nothing in. Well, this fellow had his shields well and truly up. I was not getting to him at all. I was madly thinking:

"An angle. An angle! I need an angle on this guy. I am losing him. He is already half-way back to his orthopaedic surgeon. He has one hand on the wheelchair."[41]

Then I realised:

"Truck driving! This guy is a bloody truck driver! Of course! Trucks! That's it! I'll talk about trucks. Yes!"

I began the next sentence with absolutely no idea how I would finish it, but by the time I realised I hadn't actually thought of anything more than an area of common interest and knowledge, I was committed. It went like this:

LM: "Look Bruce, it is just like driving a truck"

With that, Bruce's eyes locked in. His posture changed. He shifted a little in his seat, so that he could face me square-on. I reckon his chest puffed up just a fraction. 'Here he comes' I thought to myself. I then thought 'Sheezamageeza – what can I say now?' I went flying back in time to my stints behind the wheel, to the things

---

41 Catastrophising (awfulising): OK OK OK this *was* a bit catastrophic – perhaps I wasn't quite *this* concerned.

that used to annoy me, to my experiences and then it hit me in the face like a wiper blade on a grasshopper:

LM: "Hino's! Hino's Bruce! You know how Hino's have dodgy electronics?"

I had him. He was all of a sudden in *his* world, on *his* turf. It was as though he had *arrived*, like he had taken off his '80s beige velour tracksuit to reveal a genuinely funky pair of Nike runners. I went on:

LM: "Yeah, you know the Hino's Bruce! You know their electronics! Well, what is happening inside your nervous system is a bit like what happens sometimes in a Hino's electronics. Imagine this – you know what it's like, the fuel filter light comes on, on your dash. You think 'the fuel filter light is on, there must be something wrong with the fuel filter'. Now, this is a very sensible thing to think and it is exactly why vehicles have lights on the their dash. So, you take the truck into the mechanics and you tell him, plain and true 'there is something wrong with the fuel filter'. The mechanic looks at you as though you have just told him you're part human, part desert wilderberry, and says 'how d'yer know?' to which you reply with 'the bloody fuel filter light is on'.

That is how you knew there was something wrong in your back. There are detectors in your back that are activated when something is in danger and they send the electrical signal to your brain. It is a bit like a light coming on in your brain saying 'yep, something wrong down there, better check it out'. The reason you know

100

something has happened in your back is that your brain makes your back <u>hurt</u>.

Bruce was still with me. I pushed on.

LM: *"So, the mechanic says 'OK I'll take a look at it for you' and sure enough there is a bit of bock stuck in the fuel filter. He flushes it out. He tells you 'no worries now mate – the boys flushed it out and it looks pretty good. You should be right now.' So, you settle the bill, jump in, start it up and head back to work. No sooner than you are out on the main drag than 'Pling!', on comes the fuel filter light again. You figure that whatever was wrong with the fuel filter has obviously not been fixed and you take it back. You explain to the mechanic that there is still something wrong there and he gives you that half-vacant stare and says again 'How d'yer know?' You answer with 'because the bloody light is still bloody on!' He looks a bit surprised (which is not at all comforting – doesn't this guy know what he is doing?) and says he will take another look. This time when you pick it up, he says to you 'there may have been a little kink in the jubby winder as it comes into the top socket of the filter. We have smoothed that out, resealed it and stuck a new widget in there. Should be right as rain.' Again you settle the bill, jump in the cab, start it up and head back to work. Not long into the day you notice the same light is coming on again, intermittently at first, but then it just sits on and you think 'Shit. Bloody fuel filter.'*

Bruce: *"Too right I would – that's gotta get your blood boiling that does.*

LM: *"...so you take the truck in <u>again</u>. This time the mechanic takes the fuel filter out completely and replaces* *it with a brand new one, new pipes, <u>brand new</u> jubby winder. He shows you what he did and assures you that your truck is now 'as good as (expletive) new!' You figure it must be right now because that was a major overhaul, and it was bloody expensive. Again, (you mortgage your house) to settle the bill, jump in the cab, start it up and head back to work. Sure enough, a day in, on comes the fuel light. See Bruce, the thing with the Hino is-"*

Bruce: "It's the electronics! There must be something wrong with the electronics!"

He had it! He got it. My story had connected with something, engaged Bruce in *his* world, in *his* language, in *his domain*. It felt great, the whole group had enjoyed the story. The whole group could see Bruce as something other than *a pain patient*, something other than an overweight belligerent and whinging bludger. They started to see Bruce as some<u>one</u>. They looked at him differently, as though they were thinking 'Hang-on! Bruce is a truck driver'. In my view, these realisations are important, not just for Bruce, but for the whole group. Patients become people again, to themselves and to each other and to me. I reckon that *people* have stories and experiences that they can draw upon when they need to, but *patients* only have stories that reinforce their patient-ness. I reckon that *patients* tend to be defined by their pain, their disability and the toll and inconvenience they feel they are putting on other people. *People* don't.

I was cock-a-hoot. So I went on. The mere formality of relating this back to sensitisation of nociceptive networks would now be a cinch:

LM: "Exactly! Exactly! There must be something wrong with the electronics! The thing is Bruce, there is probably something wrong with the electronics inside you, and inside Dimos, and inside Shiela and Roberto and any human who has pain for as long as you guys have had it. Human 'electronics' change when pain persists. That is just how we are set-up – part of being a human. The system of nerves that take the danger message from the part of your body that was in danger, to your brain, becomes more sensitive. There are several ways that this happens and, unlike the truck, it is a completely normal thing for the system to become more sensitive. So, now, when the light on the dash comes on, that is, when your back hurts, it is due at least in part to the faulty electronics. You probably had an inkling for this anyway – you would do something that seemed really really minor and your back pain went through the roof. In those situations, the system is telling your brain that your back is in danger, when it probably isn't. It's just dodgy electronics. Just like the Hino."

Bruce was nodding his head and he had a faint 'ahaa' look on his face. It was like he had realised the answer to something that had been bothering him for years. I could almost hear the inner workings of his mind saying things like 'so *that's* why my back hurts when I see someone else pick up a big box'[42]. I was over the moon – I had him, I *had* him. He looked at me, still nodding and constructing his 'concluding remark'. I was ready for it – the climax of the educative process – the enlightenment – the victory!

---

42 Empathy: There is actually good evidence that we all activate parts of our brain that are involved in pain, the so-called 'pain matrix' when we see someone else being injured. Scientists call it the 'neural correlate of empathy'. If the network of neurones in the brain that produce pain are sensitised (this happens in persistent pain), then this empathy response will be greater, possibly great enough to produce pain. Take a look at the reference list because there are some good books on how the pain systems become more sensitive.

Bruce: "Yeah. I get it – I will never, <u>ever</u> buy a Hino!"

Classic. There I was, basking in the sunlight of my own canniness, feeling the warm glow of self-satisfaction, and Bruce dumped a bucket of freezing cold back-to-reality water over me.

I don't think he was joking. I think he missed it completely. Actually, it seems *I* missed it completely.

so, what on earth has the Hino story got to with pain?

I think there are two points to that story.

First, despite the spectacular failure of that metaphor with Bruce, I like it and I have used it numerous times since that one, with far better adhesion. It seems a 'sticky' story – one with which patients engage and it seems to fit the common understanding of electronics in general. Men seem to be particularly receptive to it.

Second, I sometimes reckon we learn more from our failures than our successes. I have had heaps of failures. There have been numerous times that I have busted my gut and tried and tried to give patients a handle on modern concepts of pain biology and I have not made a dent on the patients' ideas about what is going on. At first I found those sort of situations really demoralising, really deflating. I find them far less demoralising now because I think that some people are simply not ready for the information – even if you took their brain out, drip filtered in the **Textbook of Pain**, and put it back in, they mightn't get on board.

My experience with Bruce reminds me that just because I might be sitting there rating myself and rating what I am saying, it doesn't mean that the patient is.

104

references & further reading

This book is not meant to be a referenced-to-bits type of thing, obviously. Here are the references that are cited in the text, all six of them:

1.   Butler, D. & Moseley, G. L. *Explain Pain* (NOI Group Publishing, Adelaide, 2003).

2.   Adelson, E. in The new cognitive neurosciences (ed. Gazzaniga, M. S.) 339-351 (MIT Press, Cambridge, MA, 2000).

3.   Philipsen, D. Consumer age affects response to sensory characteristics of a cherry flavored beverage. J Food Sci 60, 364-368 (1995).

4.   Wall, P. Pain. The science of suffering (Orion Publishing, London, 1999).

5.   Bayer, T. L., Baer, P. E. & Early, C. Situational and psychophysiological factors in psychologically induced pain. Pain 44, 45-50. (1991).

6.   Sapolsky, R. M. Why zebras don't get ulcers: an updated guide to stress, stress-related diseases, and coping. (W.H. Freeman and Co, New York, 1998).

Now, some other stuff

The idea of this book is to get down on paper some of the stories I use to *Explain Pain* biology. It is not a textbook. No kidding Sherlock! I would like to finish this by iterating that stories and metaphors seem to be a terrific way to get at patients – to engage them with the information you are trying to get across. Modern pain biology can seem tricky if one is coming at it from a structural-pathology understanding of pain. By that I mean, an understanding of pain in which pain provides an accurate indication of the state of the tissues, which it doesn't. I believe, on the basis of what I consider to be very good evidence, that it is more accurate to say that pain provides a conscious correlate of the brain's implicit perception of threat to body tissues. I have already recommended some papers that talk about this with slightly more sophistication, in the chapter called the thirsty idiots.

I think it is important that if you are going to *Explain Pain* biology, that you actually understand it yourself. This way, you will find your own stories and metaphors and will be able to fit your stories to your patients and tell them in a way that plays to your strengths. In regards to this, I love being reminded that we each have strengths and preferred ways of working. This is exemplified in a terrific children's book called **Giraffes Can't Dance** (Andreae, G &

Parker-Rees, G (2000) Orchard Books, London). It tells the story of a giraffe called Gerald who gets despondent at the fact that he is all legs, so to speak. However, he eventually learns to dance a whole new dance. A completely original set of moves. Moves that play to his gangly strengths. My kiddies love the story almost as much as I do. I love it because it reminds me that we don't have to *Explain Pain* like Lorimer does, or like David Butler does, or like Louis Gifford does, or like anyone else does. We can explain it in our own way. Go on, be creative.

So, back to understanding it before you try and pass it on. I think that the best place to learn pain is in *Explain Pain*. *Explain Pain* is a picture book that is full of referenced research findings, but is written in a way that patients and clinicians can access it. Ideally, this book 'goes with' that one. There are other places to learn stuff about pain. Here is a list of different types of references:

Explain Pain, Butler, DS & Moseley, GL 2003 Noigroup publications, Adelaide. I think you should buy this. Go to www.noigroup.com to find out where you can buy it. If you live in the UK, you can go to www.physiouk.co.uk

Pain. The science of suffering. Wall, P. 1999. Orion Publishing, London. I was going to put a quote from me on the back of this book, just as a gag, but I got too many real ones from famous people. My own quote *would have said* that painful yarns is the most readable pain book ever, or something to that effect. That would have been a lie because *The science of suffering* remains the gold standard in pain books. Buy it.

The *Topical issues in pain* series. By CNS press (Louis Gifford). Louis knows a great deal about pain and played a key part in getting me interested in it. Thanks Louis. He is a physiotherapist and he edits a book on issues about pain that are, well, topical, to clinicians. Much of it is written at the high-end level, so it is really aimed at people who are 'into pain'. The Topical Issues series is a great place to get the state of the art in different areas of pain management and understanding. It is great value. It is endorsed by the Physiotherapy Pain Association. Go to www.achesandpainsonline.co.uk

The *Sensitive Nervous System*, Butler DS 2001 Noigroup publications, Adelaide. This was a veritable tome of all things pain biology-related. It is a few years old now so I guess there is room for an update, should David find a spare nanosecond in his life to do one. That said, I think 'SNS' remains a really good source of information. A real strength in my view is that it suggests ways to integrate the scientific data into clinical reasoning.

Wall & Melzack's Textbook of Pain. [Editors McMahon, SB & Koltzenburg, M] 2006, Elsevier, London. Now in its 5th edition, this remains the bible. However, it is serious science so put your best brain in before you try this one.

Pain, a textbook for therapists [Editors Strong, J et al] 2001, Elsevier, Edinburgh. This is a pretty occupational therapy-centric book that is aimed at allied health professionals. I have the inside word that the next edition will be far less OT-centric and include stuff from some of the key thinkers in pain from across allied health. So, the 2nd edition will be a great resource.

If you want to look at research studies that have explicitly targeted the explanation of pain biology as a treatment strategy, then here is a list of studies that I have done (I actually delivered the education for the first one, but not for any of the others):

1.   Moseley, GL [2005] Widespread brain activity during an abdominal task is markedly reduced by pain physiology education – fMRI evaluation of a patient with

chronic low back pain. Aus J Physioth 51 49-52

2.   Moseley, GL, Nicholas, MK and Hodges, PW (2004) A randomized controlled trial of intensive neurophysiology education in chronic low back pain. Clin J Pain 20(5):324-30

3.   Moseley, GL (2002) Evidence for a direct relationship between normalisation of pain cognitions and improvement in physical performance in people with chronic low back pain after intensive education. Eur J Pain 8,1: 39-45

4.   Moseley GL (2003) Unravelling the barriers to reconceptualisation of the problem in chronic pain: The actual and perceived ability of patients and health professionals to understand the neurophysiology. J Pain 4(4) 184-189

5.   Moseley, GL (2003) Joining forces – combining cognition-targeted motor control training with group or individual pain physiology education: A successful treatment for chronic low back pain. J Man Manip Ther 11, 88-94

6.   Moseley, GL (2002) Combined physiotherapy and education is efficacious for chronic low back pain. Aus J Physioth 48, 297-302

I know that there are other research groups looking at different applications of explaining pain, the effects in different settings and with different types of patients, but nothing I know of is published yet.

post-script: call for stories

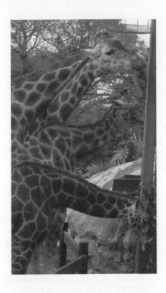

In this book, the first edition of *painful yarns*, I have attempted to record the metaphors and stories that I have found particularly helpful in explaining pain. In subsequent editions, I would like to include those metaphors and stories that other clinicians and patients have found helpful. So, consider this an official call for stories, metaphors or any other mechanisms that you use to help *Explain Pain*. I am going to run a little competition called *"The Gerald Award"*. The Gerald Award will go to the author of the submission considered by the judges to be truly excellent. There is no rule that there can only being one winner of the Gerald Award nor that you have to be a clinician, or a patient or anything in particular. This competition is so *splendidly* unregulated that you could even be related to me, the publishers and distributors, _and_ their affiliates. It will all come down to the judges' decision. The winning submission (or submissions) will be published in the next edition of _painful yarns_. A portion of royalties will be allocated to the author of the winning submission, such that they will receive about 2p for every copy of Painful Yarns that is sold. So, if your submission is good enough, you really could make an absolute motza!

Remember that the judges' decision is final and the judges are:

- Me

- A mystery pain science guru or two

- A quasi-psuedo-cluster-block randomly selected group of five people who suffer from chronic pain and who have never heard about how pain actually works.

So, send me your stories......

www.painfulyarns.com

---

* yarn:\\'yärn\\, _noun,_ a tale, especially a story of adventure or incredible happenings <He told a ripping good yarn>

In _painful yarns_, the names of some people & places have been changed to protect them from offense and me from prosecution! All the stories are based on true happenings. Like all yarns, however, the degree to which they stick to the facts is somewhat variable. In the words of Ben "Chow Mein" Hopkins, a dear friend and great story-teller, "Why ruin a really good yarn by sticking completely to the truth?"

about the author

Lorimer Moseley's first name is Graham, which is his dad's name. Lorimer is rather fond of his dad, which is why he sneaks the little 'G' in before Lorimer, which is Lorimer's mum's name and the name by which he has always been known. By sneaking the G in, Lorimer doesn't get confused with all the other Lorimer Moseley's out there.

Lorimer graduated from the University of Sydney with an Honours degree in Physiotherapy. He then decided to be a musician. This was a daft decision & he would have starved if he didn't eventually accept a job as a physiotherapist. To his surprise, he quite enjoyed being a physiotherapist. He was a physiotherapist at the New South Wales Academy of Sport for several years, then at the (Sydney) University Clinic for several years. He then undertook a PhD at the Pain Management Research Institute, Faculty of Medicine, University of Sydney. His supervisors were Prof Paul 'The walking cortex' Hodges, and A/Prof Michael 'Mr CBT' Nicholas. He gained a National Health & Medical Research Council Post-doctoral fellowship, first at the University of Queensland and then at the University of Sydney. Now he works at Oxford University in the UK, where he is Nuffield Medical Research Fellow in the Department of Physiology, Anatomy & Genetics. He lives with his family an eight-minute fast-cycle away from work, next to the Port Meadow, on which they fly the kite & take regular strolls.

Lorimer's previous book, co-authored with David 'Pain Science' Butler, is **Explain Pain**. It is a real hit with clinicians, researchers & patients. The American Pain Society Review said **Explain Pain** should be in every clinician's library! Lorimer agrees. So of course, should **painful yarns**. Lorimer's experimental & clinical research has received international awards, including: Best Paper, at the World Congress of Physical Therapy, the Cardon Award for Excellence in a Published Research Study & the Elsevier Award for Rehabilitation Research. Lorimer is author of 50 peer-reviewed publications on pain science & pain management. Elsevier Publishing assure him that his new book, '**Pain. A different kind of textbook**' will be available in early 2008.

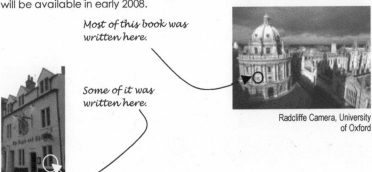

Most of this book was written here.

Some of it was written here.

Radcliffe Camera, University of Oxford

The Eagle & Child, St Giles, Oxford